AUTISM 2 AWESOME

AUTISM 2 AWESOME

ALLOW YOUR GREATEST CRISIS TO
BECOME YOUR GREATEST MIRACLE

KERRY L. BROOKS

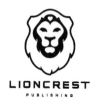

LIONCREST
PUBLISHING

AUTISM 2 AWESOME
Allow Your Greatest Crisis to Become Your Greatest Miracle

ISBN   978-1-5445-1546-5 *Hardcover*
       978-1-5445-1545-8 *Paperback*
       978-1-5445-1544-1 *Ebook*

CONTENTS

In my life, there was no light, only darkness. Once upon a time, there was joy. Now, there was only pain. My laughter had turned into sadness. Tears of happier times flowed into the river of despair. I was slowly drowning and falling into hopelessness. I cried out, "Dear God, why me?" and a quiet voice whispered back, "Why not you?"

Autism 2 Awesome:
I PROMISE.
I promise as a father, mother, sister, or brother
To love our children
Like no other
I promise as grandparents to lend a hand
As we help
Our grandchildren's knowledge expands
I promise as a teacher to use the best teaching techniques
And guide our children
Who are special and unique
I promise as a friend to help with the struggle,
Because these children
Are our sisters and brothers
I promise to help as a neighbor
Whenever you ask me
for a favor
I promise to teach tolerance and respect
To other people
Who autism does not affect
I PROMISE

INTRODUCTION

When our son Max was three years old, he was diagnosed with autism. Our primary physician at that time told us to give up on our son, because there was nothing we could do for him. He told us to prepare him for a group home and focus on having other children.

After hearing these words, I was stressed, depressed, and a total mess. The old me immediately shouted to the doctor, "How ignorant of you!" The new me would thank him if I ever saw him again. I actually said, "As my doctor, this is the best advice that you have about my son?" I informed him that our family no longer needed his services. He proved to me that people can only teach you what they know—and he didn't know anything about autism, perseverance, attitude, and a host of other life strategies I've learned since that day.

That doctor's pessimism and misinformation set me on a path of discovery that brought me face-to-face with my greatest fears and led me to overcome my greatest challenges.

During the writing of my journey, our son graduated with

honors from high school. He was also accepted into the one university that he applied to and earned a scholarship to attend.

LEAVE NO STONE UNTURNED

Allow me to start with my life's greatest crisis because that is exactly what I was going through. That's what I imagine we all go through when we hear those words for the very first time: "Your child has autism."

His mom and I instinctively responded, "What is autism?"

If I were dying of thirst, where would I look for drinking water? Everywhere. After Max's diagnosis, I was dying of thirst for knowledge about autism and answers about how to help our son. I didn't understand what autism was or how it could happen to our family.

I asked myself, "If I don't understand this diagnosis, how am I going to help Max?" Maybe you've had similar questions and searched for answers. As a family, we felt isolated, and as a father, I felt that I had let my child down. We were the abnormal family that people whispered about. Our world had changed forever.

I started to look under every stone for answers. The following is what I learned from my research (and the rest of this book is based on my years of experience as the father of an AWESOME little boy—who happens to have autism).

The information below was gathered from the website of the World Health Organization (WHO):

Autism spectrum disorder (ASD) refers to a range of conditions characterized by some degree of impaired social behavior, communication and language, and a narrow range of interests and activities that are both unique to the individual and carried out repetitively. ASDs begin in childhood and tend to persist into adolescence and adulthood. In most cases the conditions are apparent during the first 5 years of life.

You can also find additional information regarding autism on the website of the Centers for Disease Control and Prevention (CDC): www.cdc.gov/ncbddd/autism/facts.html.

WHAT WE NOTICED

When Max was about two and a half or three years old, we started to notice him displaying some curious behavior. We first became concerned when his normal vocabulary regressed to only two words. Then, he began having long, drawn-out meltdowns that occurred multiple times during the day. They seemed to last forever. We noticed he was very sensitive to loud sounds and developed an aversion to certain smells. He had serious trouble sleeping through the night. For some reason, he loved to crawl under the bed and into tight spaces, and he'd stare at his toys for as long as you would allow him to do so.

We also discovered the hard way that he was allergic to certain foods, which would cause irritability and hyperactivity, and he only wanted to eat certain foods. He was fixated on his routines, and disrupting them led to many of the well-dramatized meltdowns. All of these realizations were scary, but we forged ahead and helped him meet many milestones. Now, many years later, I know we are better people today than we were before the journey began.

MISCONCEPTIONS ABOUT AUTISM

Before our own child receives a diagnosis, we think autism is something that happens to other families. When the disorder doesn't personally affect us, it's easy to think something must be wrong with the parents, that all the child really needs is some good discipline, or that their mother didn't show them love. What a total misconception.

Another misconception among parents whose children don't have special needs relates to the degree of difficulty. As parents raising a child with special needs, we all have self-doubt and wonder if we're making the right choices. We feel emotional stress and ask, "Why my child?" We worry ourselves sick about whether they will ever make any friends or be invited to a birthday party. And when our child has a birthday party and no classmates show up, all we can do is cry, because the world seems so unfair.

If your child has special needs, most of your days are likely filled with driving to doctor visits and pursuing therapies, hoping to find a flicker of light at the end of the tunnel. The experience is extremely difficult and painful. Facing the financial burden of paying for additional testing or purchasing special food and supplements, we wonder to ourselves whether we'll make it to another day. It is an unimaginably stressful life, and that, my friend, is no misconception.

One of the biggest misconceptions is that our kids can't learn. It's a BIG misconception, because in fact, they can and do learn. They just do so in a different way, and we have to find out how they can best reach their full potential.

IT'S NOT AN EASY ROAD

Life before Max was born—when I had only myself to care for—was so much simpler.

A year or two before he was born, I was living in Nicosia, Cyprus, and—as they say on the island—life was good. People come from all over the world to vacation there and enjoy the beautiful beaches, amazing food, and hospitality of the local people. I was fortunate enough to be selected to serve there as a United States diplomat. Life in Cyprus was a wonderful opportunity to experience a new culture, new people, different food, a new language, and different ideas. I quickly learned to embrace it all.

Oh, I was having a good time. Imagine a young man experiencing his first overseas assignment. I sat at the round table with the U.S. ambassador and other heads of agencies. I had the pleasure of meeting foreign dignitaries during my international career. Assignments to Lagos, Nigeria, and Guayaquil, Ecuador, would come later, with equal amounts of adventure.

I've learned life is full of adventures. Some you plan for, and the others are thrust upon you. Either way, they both consist of ups and downs that we can greet as a crisis or an opportunity.

Early one morning in November 2000, it was time; I was about to be a father. We rushed to the hospital, thinking Max would be delivered right away. About twelve hours later, he entered the world and I said to him in Greek, "Welcome to Cyprus," but I can't remember how to say it now. His birth reaffirmed to me the awesome power and goodness of God. I was amazed to be a part of something so beautiful. I knew I was blessed.

Little did I know that the greatest adventure of all was still to come.

I enjoyed being a new father, and I was learning a lot about caring for another person, including waking up all through the night to change diapers and feed him. It was crazy good. Then, I witnessed him take his first steps and heard him laugh out loud for the first time.

I remember the first time he had an ice cream cone. He took one lick, and while his brain was trying to process whether he liked it or not, his eyes danced around in his head, looking at the ice cream cone as if it were a new life form to study. I guess his brain said, "We don't know what this is, but we like it." I laughed over the bewilderment in his eyes as his brain communicated with his taste buds, "Yeah, we like this stuff. Send more, please."

BE FIRST 2 RESPOND

Since that day in 2003 when we first heard the diagnosis, I have been committed to helping improve the quality of Max's life and helping him reach his full potential. When I thought about our son, I thought about his untapped qualities and as-yet-undeveloped abilities. I thought about the contribution he would one day make to the world. I thought about him living his true purpose and reaching his fulfillment.

Developing his fundamental skills was essential for him to reach his full potential.

It would be a hard-fought battle and one that I was not prepared for. I would see our financial savings dwindle in a few months' time. There was very little me time or couple time because everything was about Max. The bills piled up higher and higher, but they had to be paid somehow.

Inspired by the journey with my son, I started a company called Autism 2 Awesome. Our life strategy is "We Train the World to Be First 2 Respond."

Max inspired the name of the company during our journey together. I knew that autism was a label, but I also knew that this label would not determine his full potential. I urgently needed to shift the perspective of our entire family. I wanted our mindset to be one of awesome experiences, gratitude, and a total appreciation for the opportunity to be here. It was my purpose to help us travel from the mindset of Autism 2 Awesome. It has been a life-changing experience.

Based on my life experiences, I wanted to teach our son to respond to a crisis as opposed to reacting. Many times when we react to a crisis, we do so out of fear, without thought, in an impulsive, emotional, and illogical way.

On the other hand, we can *respond* to a crisis, with a well-planned, creative, thoughtful, unemotional, logical, and solution-oriented mindset.

Be First 2 Respond offers life strategies that teach you to rethink, reimagine, and recondition the misconceptions about autism. Our strategies are taught using our Special Intervention Training Techniques (SITT).

In fact, Be First 2 Respond is so important that each chapter of this book is one piece of our complete life-strategy training:

Be Better Than Your Best: A crisis will accept nothing less.

Expectations: Change them and you can change your life.

First-Step Fears: We all have fears, but we can't let them stop us from taking the first steps.

Imagination without Limitations: Having a vision means you can plan for a future where the only thing stopping you is what you can think up!

Responsibility: The safety and security of your family is up to you—and only you are responsible for your miracles.

Systems of Routines: Find what works for you and use it—again and again.

Teamwork: It's always better when we can work together.

Resilience: Get it and use it, and you can get through anything.

Exposure & Experiences: The more exposure to new experiences you and your family have, the more you learn from them.

Special Intervention Training Techniques (SITT): Early intervention is the key to success.

Power of Prayer: Prayer is the most powerful thing I know, and you can use it as a guiding force on your journey.

One Day: Turn that "one day" you've always dreamed of into today!

Never Give Up: When parenting a child with autism, failure is not a final option.

Decide: Only one person can allow your greatest crisis to become your greatest miracle—and that's you!

When you follow these fourteen strategies, you will find remarkable success.

OUR GREATEST MIRACLE

In November 2018, Max turned eighteen years old—and he has a promising life ahead of him. He graduated with honors from the high school where he studied in Guayaquil, Ecuador.

He participated in organized sports, plays a musical instrument, learned a second language, is an excellent swimmer, and completed physics and advanced math. At the writing of this book, Max has been accepted to a university in Arizona.

Fifteen years earlier, a doctor told us to give up on our child. That doctor was ignorant, and if anyone tells you to give up on your child, then they are also ignorant.

During our family journey, I learned a lot about myself, about other people, and about what it means to live with autism. When I started to look beyond the label of autism, I discovered the most beautiful smile my son would give me from time to time. I discovered his shining blue eyes. And I discovered a human being with a kind heart, compassion, and a beautiful spirit who makes a positive impact on the world.

If you have the courage to allow your greatest crisis to become your greatest miracle, then you're ready to start your journey. Chapter 1 will show you how to be better than your best.

DOS & DON'TS

At the end of each chapter, you'll see a section called "Dos & Don'ts," where I've included some key takeaways for you to remember. Here's your first one: *don't* forget to read these!

Do learn everything you can about your child's diagnosis.

Do ask your doctor questions.

Do get ready to change your life!

Don't stop asking until you get answers.

Don't believe everything you hear about autism.

Don't turn away from this journey—you can do it!

CHAPTER ONE

BE BETTER THAN YOUR BEST

"Little children, you are from God and have overcome them, for he who is in you is greater than he who is in the world."

— I JOHN 4:4, ESV

During my lifetime, I have faced some tough challenges and a few crises that have required me to be better than my best. Trust me—it was not always easy, but it was worth it.

One of the first challenges I faced as a young man was getting accepted into college. I was academically and financially unprepared. My ACT score was so low that I am embarrassed to share it with you. Once I was accepted, I faced a new challenge: figuring out how to pay for college. I didn't have the money, my parents didn't have it, and money certainly wasn't falling out of the sky.

Later in life, I would challenge myself to complete the Disney Marathon at the age of forty-two. (Remind me not to do that again!) During my twenty-eight-year career in federal law enforcement, I would face many other challenges.

However, the greatest crisis of my life thus far was hearing that my son has autism. I found myself desperately searching for ways to help him, but I didn't know where to start.

In this chapter, I will share with you what I learned about how to be better than my best, including by dreaming of the relationship I wanted to build with my son, having the best attitude I could, being a good father, and making any adjustments necessary. Additionally, I engaged in a lot of self-reflection, kept a journal, and looked beyond what I was experiencing at the time.

Using the tools available to you and striving to be better than your best will allow for personal growth. The alternative is a lack of development. Without self-reflection to ensure you're on the right path, you may find yourself asking, "What am I doing wrong?"

A DREAM RELATIONSHIP

I have always dreamed of being a good father.

I didn't have the best relationship with my father when I was growing up. We didn't share the bond that I wanted to have with my son or develop the great two-way communication channel that I think is so important between children and their parents. Although I didn't receive the best blueprint for being a good father, I did learn other valuable lessons from him. Having a child diagnosed with autism tested my resolve and redefined my perspective of what it means to be a good father. I had to set aside my ego and put my son's well-being first. Through it all, I had to allow him to be himself—not insist on the person I was hoping he would be.

For example, I was a pretty good athlete and earned a football scholarship to play for Troy University. We even went on to win the National Championship. But I really didn't want to put expectations on my son to follow in my exact footsteps. Since I wasn't the most astute student and he faced learning challenges, I wanted him to know that with hard work, anything is possible.

I so badly wanted to give him the strategies I learned from my parents, sports, and my life's experiences.

Again, to be better than my best meant putting his needs first. I came to understand that taking care of myself and educating myself about autism would benefit him—and our entire family.

Many nights, my family and I were awake until the wee hours of the morning. I had to go to work the next day and perform on little sleep. I quickly learned that there were three things I could control, even on the most challenging days: my attitude, my self-reflection, and keeping a journal so I could see how far we'd come.

ATTITUDE

After we received the diagnosis about Max's autism, our family did not have a good attitude about our circumstances. We blamed each other, the medical field, and whomever or whatever else we could.

It soon became clear this attitude was not going to help our son's situation. In fact, our negative attitude was making life even worse for our son and ourselves. If we wanted to be better than our best so we could help our son, we had to change.

Here is what Charles Swindoll says about attitude:

The longer I live, the more I realize the impact of attitude on life. Attitude, to me, is more important than facts. It is more important than the past, than education, than money, than circumstances, than failures, than successes, than what other people think or say or do. It is more important than appearance, giftedness, or skill. It will make or break a company, a church, or a home. The remarkable thing is that we have a choice every day regarding the attitude we will embrace for that day. We cannot change our past. Nor can we change the fact that people will act in a certain way. We also cannot change the inevitable. The only thing we can do is play on the one string we have, and that is our attitude. I am convinced that life is 10 percent what happens to me and 90 percent how I react to it. And so it is with you—we are in charge of our attitudes.

When I was just a little boy playing baseball in the summer, I had all the talent in the world, but I had a bad attitude. One day while we were practicing, I was using the coach's glove. I became upset over something that I don't even remember and, in my anger, took off the glove, threw it into the air, and walked off the field. After practice, the coach drove my brother and me home. To my surprise, he spoke to my mother about the little incident. After he left, my mother told me, "If you don't change your attitude and listen to the coach, then you are off the baseball team." I was shocked. It was summer, and I played baseball every summer! I loved the sport, but my career was about to be over because of my attitude.

That night, I wrote a note to my mother begging her to let me continue playing on the team—and I promised her that I would change my attitude.

I learned a valuable lesson about attitude early on. Because of my mother's discipline, I changed. I became a better team player, and I eventually used my positive attitude and talents to earn that football scholarship and help win the championship.

I recently told this story to a colleague of mine, and he was amazed that I was part of a National Championship. After hearing my story, he commented to me, "You will always be a winner."

I just chuckled. Later, I thought about his comment and acknowledged he was right. I *will* always be a winner. See, I believe that when we give our all, especially to our children with special needs, we can all be winners. We pass this attitude forward to our children.

AN ADJUSTMENT

One of the lessons I learned during my journey is when I had a negative attitude, I had low expectations for my life. (We will discuss expectations later in the book.)

When people have a bad attitude, they tend to focus on the obstacles. They don't realize those obstacles are only temporary and actually offer the opportunity to make us stronger and wiser. People with bad attitudes usually think of themselves and influence others in a negative way. Look at where you are today and ask yourself, "Could my life be better if I had the right attitude?"

Could you have a greater positive impact on your child if you had the right attitude? Attitude is one of those few things in life that you have complete control over. Only you are responsible for your attitude.

Long ago, I stopped blaming others for Max's diagnosis—and I stopped blaming myself as well. As a result, I was able to see all the good I already had in my life. I had a beautiful son with a gifted mind, and I wanted to discover how to help him develop those gifts. I had the opportunity to be a part of something special that was bigger than me. I had the opportunity right in front of me to unlock a gifted young mind that would later go on and positively impact humanity.

At his high school, all the teachers comment on his exceptional manners and kindness to others. Imagine what the world would be like if we all shared our gift of kindness. They comment on the thought-provoking questions he asks during class discussion. When we discuss his college career, he always talks about studying a curriculum that will help others have a better experience in life.

We all have gifts to share with others, if only to make the world just a little bit better place. I also believe when we share our gifts, we benefit as the giver. I learned so much from helping my son, and I want to share my knowledge to help you.

It's amazing to see the transformation the right attitude brings. As a family, we started attracting people into our lives—doctors, teachers, conferences, and impactful information—by having the right attitude. I found I was more focused on the solution than the problem. I also helped our son to discover his purpose, well-being, and happiness—without comparing him to other children.

When I discovered the right attitude, I was able to see the light and not live in the darkness.

I didn't ask for this crisis, but it was necessary to bring me where

I am today. I believe that with the right attitude, we are unstoppable—because I have lived it, experienced it, and witnessed it. There is something awesome about having the right attitude. People around you will start to change theirs as well. They'll see your disposition in life and want some of it for themselves.

I'm not telling you it's going to be easy to have the right attitude, but it will be worth it. You will understand that hard times don't always last and failure is just another stepping stone to success. We discovered as a family that the person with the right attitude understands we are committed to a higher and greater purpose than ourselves—one that, for whatever reason, has been entrusted to us. We're responsible for seeing it through.

Our son inherently trusted us with his life, and we only had one opportunity to get it right. Doing so required the right attitude. So if you care to change your world, start with the right attitude, because then you can never lose. Life is 10 percent what happens to us and 90 percent how we respond to it.

Today, our son is an adult—and I am awestruck by his awesome attitude. Teachers at his school always comment about him is a positive way. I like to think that as parents, we played a small role in his great outlook.

SELF-REFLECTION

Along our journey, I also learned that to be better than my best I had to be open to self-reflection.

Self-reflection is taking the opportunity to look at yourself from within. There are always events happening in the world that can have a positive or negative impact on our lives. It's important to ask, "How am I responding to everything going on in my life, and how is it impacting me?"

Self-reflection is a time to look within and observe, not judge yourself regarding how you should or shouldn't respond to external circumstances. If you are able to respond to a situation without negative emotions, then you can have less anxiety, less stress, lower blood pressure, and better sleep. You can enjoy a more purpose-filled life. You will also be more useful to your child and the situation you are going through.

When my life is going well, I rarely take the time for self-reflection. Why would I need to, right? If things are going well, then I must be doing everything right!

Wrong.

I will say this: I think self-reflection is easier when life is going well, because we are more open and less susceptible to a pre-judgment mentality. When things are going well and I take the time for self-reflection, my thoughts are clear and I can have a positive inner dialogue that helps me continue with the good times. I also learn how to handle a crisis a little better.

I don't think anybody wants to go through a crisis. And somehow, they always come at the worst time in your life. I have never heard a person say, "I wish I had a crisis going on in my life."

I can attest—and so can you—that going through a crisis is tough. You feel like you won't make it through, but you can. And you can come out of it stronger. When our son was diagnosed with autism, I felt so helpless and afraid that I thought I would die. I felt sorry for him, because I was not better prepared to help him through his most difficult time.

I thought, *Why does this have to happen right now?*

I started to self-reflect, and it was all negative. I could only see the darkness and not the light. I didn't want to reflect; I wanted someone to tell me how to fix my child—as if he were a broken toy.

Looking back now, I realize there was nothing to fix. Life gave me just what I needed at that particular time, even though I didn't recall asking for it, nor did I want it. It was going to be so damn hard. Life doesn't care.

I wasn't where I wanted to be. However, I was where I was at the moment—and I wouldn't be there forever. I realized that I couldn't control external forces. I had to look deep inside myself and find the sliver of light that could lead me out of this dark place.

The dark place I'm referring to is not Max's diagnosis but rather the negative outlook that society has for children with autism. I had to reflect and not allow myself to buy into the bullshit of society. Through self-reflection, I was able to wash off the stench of what the rest of the world thought about children like my son. I was able to see and feel the small but growing flame burning inside of me to find a way to help my son live his purpose.

We all have a purpose, and self-reflection allows us to tap into something that we might not have known was there.

I knew Max was a diamond, but how could I help him shine? I

remember one of my first aha moments with him. I was chasing him through the house with an oversized exercise ball, saying, "I'm gonna getchu," in a silly voice. He laughed and continued to run. I circled back around and waited for him to run right into this giant exercise ball. Then, he would bounce off of it and laugh, before taking off running again in the other direction.

In the middle of the chase, I stopped and waited for him to make his next move. I noticed that he had also stopped and was waiting for me to make my next move. When I came around the corner, he saw which direction I was coming from and took off running the other way.

I was stunned. Max had used his senses, his patience, and his intellect to evaluate my plans. I looked at his mother and shouted to her, "Did you see that?"

I learned that day that his brain worked perfectly, but it worked differently from those of other people. From that day on, I knew exactly how I would train him to reach his purpose and best potential. And along the way, he taught me so much more and helped me to discover my real purpose.

Self-reflection taught me to stay engaged with my son even if I didn't have all the answers. I reflected on how I could be better than my best, and the answers always came. Once I felt the flame burning inside of me, there was no stopping me from being the very best dad I could be for my son!

KEEP A JOURNAL

When I am in the process of self-reflecting and changing my attitude, there are a lot of emotions swirling inside of me. I started keeping a journal of my thoughts, events, progress, feelings, and whatever else I wanted to record.

I also added my reasons for gratitude, because I believe that the more thankful you are, the more you realize how much you have. Taking the time to sit down and write out my gratitude was my way of acknowledging my appreciation of the many blessings I already had and the many to come.

One of the first times we started keeping a journal was for our son. There was so much information coming our way that we could not remember it all. We were reading books about autism, traveling to conferences, trying different treatment programs, and discussing the newfound information with each other.

As a family, we worked together to track his progress, which proved highly beneficial every time we had a doctor appointment. Most of the doctors give you about fifteen minutes at each appointment to give them your child's complete medical history. By keeping this journal, we had the most important facts available to tell the doctor about Max.

The journal allowed us to review his life whenever we wanted to. We tracked his progress, how many temper tantrums he had, his food allergies, how many hours he was sleeping, and even the color, smell, and consistency of his poop—yes, we kept track of everything. We had a complete picture of our son's life written down for review.

To become better than our best, we had to dedicate ourselves to him. When we started keeping journals, we discovered so much more than we could have ever retained with our memory alone.

By keeping a journal, you will have your life story at your fingertips, allowing you to become better than your best each day if you so choose.

I still write my thoughts down on a regular basis. This process has allowed me to review the past through my own words, which helps me to appreciate where I am now. Looking back, some of the things I wrote in my journal sounded like they came from someone who does not resemble how I see myself. I was able to be myself in my journal without any internal or external judgment, express my greatest fears without being fearful, and grow stronger because I took a good look at myself from the inside. There are not many people who know exactly what our son went through and how far he has come—but I do, because I was there every step of the way.

Every day, I do my best to remind him how much I love him and how proud of him I am. The journey with him made me a better person, and I hope his journey with me added a little flavor to his life.

Keeping a journal resulted in my writing a children's book, *Daddy & Me*. It also led me to write and record eight children's songs. By keeping a journal, we were able to see the path we had traveled. Better yet, we were able to have a guide to look beyond where we were at that moment.

LOOK BEYOND

It's hard to overcome a crisis, but it's not impossible. People do it every day in their own way and in their own time.

When I was going through my most difficult times with my son,

I had to look beyond the problems of the day and think about all the possibilities outside my current experience. I held the vision of my son living a purpose-filled life that included happiness and good health. I didn't focus so much on whether he was keeping up academically with other kids his age. I wanted him to be happy and healthy, and to do his best while I did my best for him. We all have talents, but we don't all have the same talents—and that's what makes us different, unique, and special parts of this beautiful world.

When I looked beyond the label of autism, I could enjoy this beautiful angel who would teach me how to appreciate life and to be thankful for the blessing that God has given each of us. I was supposed to be helping him, but he helps me to be better than my best every day.

If not for the journey that I experienced with my son, I would not be here sharing this book with you. Within each of us, we have the ability to look beyond and chart the future that we want to experience.

Once I began to look beyond, I started to notice miracles happening in my life. Or maybe the miracles were always there, but I didn't see them because I was focused on something else. Our family discovered the right doctors for our son at the right stage of life. In school, the right teachers started to appear to teach him, and there would always be some email with information coming in that seemed to be right on time.

What do you see when you look beyond the label of autism? Can you see the growth that you and your family have made together? Can you see the possibilities of tomorrow? Can you allow your blessings and miracles to appear?

Whatever you see, write it in your journal and start being a better you and living a more purposeful life. I challenge you to look beyond wherever you are in life and allow your greatest crisis to become your greatest miracle.

Looking beyond has blessed me long after I traveled through the most difficult days with my son. Today, I am grateful that our journey together has taught me to look beyond and see possibilities that others cannot see for me. I am grateful he blessed me with a monumental challenge that would help me strive to be better than my best.

During the writing of my book, I asked my sister-in-law Nacoal, who is a hero of a mother to a son on the spectrum, about expectations regarding our children with autism. I asked her if she thought we should lower our expectations for children on the spectrum. She thoughtfully replied that we should *change* our expectations. I agree with her, and I find this response applicable to life in general. We all have expectations of life, but have we ever thought about what life expects of us? All of us have a purpose, and I think we must learn to change our expectations to discover it.

DOS & DON'TS

Do take time for self-reflection.

Do look beyond the diagnosis to see your child for who he or she is.

Do keep a journal and look back on how far you've come in your journey already.

Don't miss your miracles.

Don't miss making great memories.

Don't compare your child to other children.

CHAPTER TWO

CHANGE YOUR EXPECTATIONS

"A wonderful gift may not be wrapped as you expect."

—JONATHAN LOCKWOOD HUIE

Sometimes I've wished my son could just be "normal" like all the other kids. When I learned I was having a child, I had many expectations for him. Oh, I was so excited for him to play sports, and we could go out in the backyard and play catch. I expected him to be the jock athlete like me and be one of the most popular kids by his junior year of high school.

In this chapter, I'll share with you how I changed my expectations and allowed Max to be Max. I also let go of my ego, because this journey was all about his well-being, and I had to think about his best interests and how could I serve him. At the end of the day, I had to let go of my expectations if I sincerely wanted my son to make friends, live life to his true potential, and explore the world unafraid.

If I didn't change my mindset about Max, I risked him trying to live up to my expectations all his life. He would have been living in my dark shadow instead of the light of his true self. No child deserves to be smothered by this kind of pressure from their parents.

Many times, our expectations don't meet our reality. I remember when I was about to graduate from high school and I didn't know what I wanted to do with my life. I didn't have a scholarship to play my favorite sport, which was football, so my choices were very limited—or so I believed.

One day, my brother and I were passing the football back and forth in the front yard while I was dreaming of playing in the NFL. That dream was my expectation; in reality, I didn't even have a college scholarship. He mentioned to me that I could walk on (try out) at Troy University. He added that Troy had just won the Division II National Championship in football, and the school was only about an hour from his house. I felt excited about the idea, but I had questions. For one, what was a walk-on? He explained that I would have the chance to try out for Troy's football team, along with other colleges. If I was good enough, I would earn a scholarship to attend school. I seized on this adventure since I didn't have any money to pay for college, and I did exactly what he suggested.

I took my talents and my one or two suitcases and headed to Troy. When I arrived, I had to change my expectations. On my first day of practice, I received a pair of pink football pants that were supposed to be white. Our jersey color was red, and it had bled onto the white pants, so I got pink ones. All the starters had clean white pants, and I wanted a pair, too.

See, in high school, I got used to much better treatment than I received in my first days of college practice. I approached the manager (not the coach) who was handing out the pants, and I politely requested a pair of white ones. He looked at me and asked in a condescending tone, "Are you here to play football or worry about how you look?" Boy, he made me madder than a hippo with a hernia, but he was right.

I had no money for college, and I needed to make this football team so I could pay to go to school. I didn't care what I looked like. Every obstacle strengthens me for greater obstacles in life. There were a lot of talented players attempting to walk on the team who never made it, but I did.

When it came to my son, I didn't care what I had to look like in order to help him, and I didn't mind changing my expectations when I understood how doing so would help him live a more purpose-filled life.

So I changed from expecting him to grow out of autism and be "normal" like the other kids to my new reality, which was to love him right here and right now and to help him be happy, healthy, and live a purposeful life to his best potential—no matter what it looked like. I started to see how imposing preconceived notions from my childhood onto Max limited his development and growth.

BE MAX

Let me explain. Let's say Max did grow up to be a football player like me. He makes a lot of money, buys a lot of material things, and even has fame. Wow, he is just like his father. Maybe it would be less stressful for him, though, if I allowed him to have his own dreams, without my expectations. Maybe one day he owns a sports franchise or becomes a youth sports coach and teaches kids the importance of hard work, good sportsmanship, the simple joy of playing sports, and the value of discipline to achieve success.

When we change our expectations, it doesn't mean that we are *lowering* them. Change can be good. Now, change may not feel so great in the beginning, but give it some time. I know, by now you're saying, "I get that changing expectations can be good, but how do I go about doing that?" Great question—I'm so glad you asked. I will share my process with you.

LET GO OF THE EGO

I had this huge thing called an ego, and I had to learn to let it go. I am reminded of this quote by Lao Tzu:

Act without expectation.

First of all, every day I looked at the gentleness and the compassionate heart of our little boy, and I would ask how could I serve him best. Once I realized it was all about him and not about my self-serving interest, I aimed to be the best father I could. I did my best to be there for him day and night, to be honest with him, and, most importantly, to listen to him regarding his needs.

One of the first things I did was read to my son, engage with him, and encourage him to engage with me. I knew that reading with him would help increase his vocabulary and allow him to express his thoughts and feelings better. Max did not interact with us naturally, which was a huge concern to us. We always wondered how he would make friends and whether he would remain isolated in his own world. We felt scared, and I know such worries must feel scary for you as well. Imagining our child spending the rest of his life alone in his own little world brought tears to my eyes.

By reading to him, I hoped to ignite a spark of interest that would allow us to build a connection with him, one day inspiring him to use his verbal communication and speak to us. I hoped he would become interested in the world around him and start to use his creativity that was locked away inside. I wanted to motivate him to engage in more physical activities and less mind-numbing television. I practiced my strategy daily without any expectations, but I felt hopeful.

Every moment was new, and every day blessed us with opportunities to help our son. Because I did not have any expectations, new ideas flowed from me constantly and I was better able to understand my son's needs. Without expectations blocking my mind, I could fully engage him while building positive memories together. Without expectations blocking our relationship, we could just be father and son enjoying our journey together.

Reading to Max almost every night was a gateway for me to be part of his world and for him to join the rest of the world. I recalled when I was younger and preparing to graduate from college; my mother asked me what I planned to do next. I told her I was going to float and go with the flow. She laughed her head off, which made me laugh as well. But that is exactly what I did: I went with the flow, and I have been greatly surprised by life. My experiences have greatly exceeded any expectations others might have had for me. They set their expectations way too low for me based on their life experiences, and I was not going to do that to Max. I wanted him to enjoy being surprised by life.

Here is a quick story. About a month before Max graduated from high school, he had to complete his senior presentation. The morning of his presentation, he reminded me what time I needed to be at the school and I assured him I would be there. When I arrived and entered the school library where Max was about to begin his presentation, I was amazed. He was dressed in a nice suit and looked like a million bucks. At that moment, I had a flash of a vision of Max one day presenting to Fortune 500 companies about how he could help them make their products or services better. Such a vision never would have been possible if I thought he had to meet my expectations.

After Max was diagnosed with autism, I set my expectations far too low for him based on my fears as well as the fears of others who did not understand their debilitating power. By letting go of my own ego, the natural process of learning could begin to shape his development through his own curiosity, along with play, listening to music, and constant interaction.

When he was two or three years old, I'd play a game with him that I called "tickle time." I read somewhere that laughter is good medicine that boosts the immune system. So I would chase him down, pick him up, and gently toss him onto the bed, and I would start the tickle game with him. I would use my hands to tickle his tummy. When he covered his tummy, I would tickle him under his arms and then his feet.

He would be in complete heaven, and so would I, because I could see the light in his eyes and the joy and excitement in his face. I could feel the vibration of his body welcoming one of the greatest stress relievers: laughter. These were magical moments that bonded us together emotionally.

Then, in the middle of the game, I would stop and ask him to repeat the alphabet with me. I would count and ask him to repeat after me. In this way, we started to incorporate traditional learning. I think it's easier for our children to learn when they're free from the stress of expectations—the same is true for adults and professionals, too. Without any expectations, I learned how to help my child absorb and retain information in a fun, interesting, and creative way.

Oh boy, was I excited. Now, my creative juices started to flow, and I was elated to be a part of this process. At the time, I had no idea I would write a book and share this information with you and the rest of the world. At that moment, it was just between Max and me.

THE GREATER GOOD

After letting go of ego, I asked myself how each of my actions would serve him for the greater good.

Remembering my experiences as a child, I wanted to know how my decisions would impact his greater being—especially his well-being. From this perspective, I stopped comparing him to other children and stopped comparing him to myself when I was his age. Sometimes it was tempting to wonder why my son couldn't do what other kids could or be like them, but such questions were ridiculous on my part and not very useful for Max. I had to stop the comparison. It wasn't getting him or me anywhere. In fact, it added unnecessary stress to his life and made him withdraw even further. I realized I had to reduce his stress as much as possible.

Most of us have experienced the negative impact of stress on our lives. A lot of people have a tough time coping with stressful situations even as adults. Now, imagine being on the autism spectrum and having additional stress in your life because your parents, caregivers, teachers, and society want you to be just like everyone else. I was there every day watching my son struggle through life, having a difficult time coping with the stress of going to different doctors and keeping up with his classmates. Did I really want to add unrealistic parental expectations to the list of stressors?

Life can be difficult no matter who you are, but it is especially so if you're on the autism spectrum. So, I was determined to find ways to reduce the stress in his life. I knew if I could find good strategies, they would have a huge impact on his life. The reduction of stressful situations in anybody's life is going to have a positive impact. I knew that feeling less stress would probably allow him to sleep better, improve his mood, boost his immune system, help build his self-confidence, and make learning easier for him. This was by no means an easy task.

My professional job demanded a lot from me, and to be honest, my career suffered. My job expected more from me, but I was focused on the health of my son. I knew I had a limited time to do good by him and give him my total commitment, because whatever I did would impact the rest of his life. I had to go hard, and I had to be dedicated. I let all of my expectations go and provided him with unconditional love. The only thing he needed to do was just be.

He gave me unconditional love, so the least I could do was reciprocate. Our love for one another got us through a lot of tough days, but the interaction between us that followed built a bond that I never imagined possible.

Without expectations and the stress of expectations, I had the opportunity to witness the progress of his speech each and every day from the interaction that we shared. I was driven, but not driven to win—just driven to be involved and to guide him to the best of my ability. I saw my son constantly improve as I helped to reduce the stress in his life. He was able to smile more and simply be himself without the feeling of being pushed to do anything better.

END THE EXPECTATIONS

Sri Chinmoy said, "Peace begins when expectation ends." Without expectation, I did my best to help Max smile and laugh every day.

Seeing him happy made me happy. These are the times that I still cherish and carry with me. Along our journey, I discovered that when my child is smiling and laughing, there are no expectations—only enjoying and experiencing life in the moment.

You might be curious to know how to make your child laugh. Max and I used to play a game in which he'd choose a story from a book and we would act it out. I did this to help build his creativity, critical thinking, and leadership skills—and it was just fun for both of us. At this particular time in his life, he was into dragons. I knew the story well because I read it to him on a regular basis. I put him on my back, and we were on our way to go dragon hunting. He had his sword in his hands and was ready for the fight.

I was excited because he was coming out of his shell. I didn't expect this behavior from him, but I liked it. I yelled to him, "I see the dragon, so get ready!" and it became a fierce imaginary fight. I yelled, "Look out! Here comes his fire!" and made an evasive move so we wouldn't get burned up. He hung on to me tightly so he wouldn't fall off and be devoured by the dragon. I laughed, he laughed, and we both laughed some more.

I yelled to Max once more, "Get your sword ready—we have the dragon right where we want him!" I was excited that my son was about to slay the dragon. We got closer and closer, and I asked him if he was ready. He responded, "Hey, I have an idea. Why don't we tickle the dragon and make him our friend?" I never expected that idea from my son. It was so much better than I could have ever expected. So we tickled the dragon and made him our friend, and we all lived happily ever after.

Now, every child is different, but everybody loves a good game of something. The other games we played during father and son time would progress in a similar fashion. I wanted to serve my son's highest needs, and along the way, I learned to let go of my expectations. During his younger years, we passed our days together in this way. I was always thinking about helping him to be stress-free while having a blast in life. Looking back, the time passed quickly. Simply asking a couple of questions about how I could serve his highest good and ease his stress led to a chapter in my book.

From the time we spent together, I was inspired by Max to write a children's book called *Daddy & Me*. I wanted to remember those times forever, and now I can look back and relive some of those moments. Reading together helps build a strong social relationship between father and son, and you can't get a doctor's prescription for that bond.

Changing my expectations created a foundation that led to positive consequences for my son's ability to make friends, develop high self-esteem, and be unafraid to pursue new adventures in life. I didn't expect such great results. Today, I watch Max enjoying life and accomplishing things that I never thought were possible. Often, we sit and talk, and he'll tell me about his day. Then, he'll tell me about everything that he would like to accomplish after finishing high school. It's an awesome feeling, and I am so proud of him.

DOS & DON'TS

Do change expectations—yours and those of people around you.

Do listen to your child's needs.

Do allow learning to be fun!

Don't expect your child to be like others.

Don't expect your child to be like you.

Don't expect the process to be easy.

CHAPTER THREE

FIRST-STEP FEARS

"Remember your dreams and fight for them. You must know what you want from life. There is just one thing that makes your dream become impossible: the fear of failure."

—PAULO COELHO

After we were told that Max had autism, I was paralyzed with fear. I found myself no longer dreaming of a bright future for him but instead contemplating all the difficult challenges that awaited him. My mind ran wild, thinking of all kinds of bad possibilities that could hurt him. I would often think, *I am his father, and I am supposed to be able to protect him from anything—but how do I protect him from autism?* I really wanted to be a good father to him and protect him from all the bad forces in the world.

I continued to fear the worst for him, and I repeated these fearful stories over and over inside of my head. Maybe you have experienced something similar and just couldn't move forward. But we must continue to move forward if we are going to make progress. I realized that almost nothing could harm him more than my failure to face my fears.

Most of the stories we tell ourselves are simply not true, and I would eventually become just another story if I allowed my fears to control me. I believe it was Zig Ziglar who described FEAR as false evidence appearing real.

In the Bible, 1 Timothy 1:7 says, "God has not given us a spirit of fear."

In this chapter, I will share with you my FEARS and how I was able to take the first steps to overcome them. Those steps didn't make fear magically go away overnight. Little by little and slowly but surely, I was able to face them head on—and each fear that I overcame made the other ones a little less frightening.

Overcoming fear is absolutely liberating. Personally, I gained a sense of confidence in my ability to do anything. The feeling became contagious, and Max started to develop self-esteem that improved the quality of his life. Once I overcame one fear, I knew I could overcome another one.

The danger of not overcoming our fears is that we pass them on to our children. At some point, we need to challenge ourselves to move beyond worry. We should do it for our own personal growth as well as for the betterment of our children. When we are fearful all the time, we can't relax, which adds more stress to our body. Living in fear can bring on anxiety and depression, which prevent us from being better than our best. We can become better than our best by conquering our own fears and teaching our children how to conquer theirs.

In the beginning, my fears would hinder me from being my very best for Max and for myself. After almost thirty years in law enforcement, I have seen enough to develop more than my share of fears for my child's well-being. Now, I've come to realize I was fixating on false evidence appearing real. At the time, my fears seemed real to me, but then it dawned on me that they were, in fact, creating the problem.

I can vividly remember how fearful I felt when I realized that Max would one day have to travel alone. I worried myself sick about whether he'd be able to do so. I wondered who would guide him and *what if, what if, what if.* Then, I came up with a solution. When he got a little bit older, whenever he and I would travel together, I'd coach him on exactly what to do. When we entered the airport, I'd ask whether he had his passport and remind him to have it ready for the ticketing agent. When we went through security, I'd ask him whether he'd taken his computer out of his bag. I would never do these tasks for him, because he needed to learn how to do them for himself. I practiced with him over and over.

After we completed several flights together, I presented Max with the opportunity to show me what he'd learned. It was now his turn to direct us from point A to point B in the airport, regarding what we needed to do to check in and get to the gate. In this way, I prepared him to become an international traveler, and he has now flown from Guayaquil, Ecuador, to Phoenix, Arizona, and back.

I always provided him with positive feedback on what he did correctly, and I encouraged and coached him where he needed improvement.

Once, while traveling alone, he fell asleep in the airport and missed his flight. I knew he was prepared regarding how to travel and what to do in such a situation. He contacted his mother and then went to the ticketing agent for assistance in getting booked on a later flight. He had money for food, so he was happy. There is always the possibility of a misfortune taking place, but by teaching our children strategies, we prepare them for life. I had to develop a sense of trust in my own parenting skills and in the community that was helping to shape Max's young mind.

THE FEAR OF AUTISM

When I heard the word "autism" and "Max" in the same sentence, my heart dropped and I didn't realize that my worst crisis had just begun. Just the word overwhelmed my mind with first-step fears. I wasn't a doctor, and I didn't know anything about autism. Believe me when I tell you that I was scared about which steps to take next. I understand your fear because I have lived through it. I have been at the crossroads you are now approaching. I have conquered the fear that now keeps you awake.

There were no guidebooks or roadmaps to lead me step by step. At that time, most doctors couldn't agree on effective treatment. They didn't have an answer and were afraid to tell you so, and the uncertainty made the situation even worse. When the doctor told us to plan on institutionalizing Max, fear, anger, rage, and anything else you can think of took control of my rationale. But I had no fear when I told that doctor his services were no longer needed. We decided as a family that if the doctor was not solution-oriented and willing to do what was best for our child, we could do without him. I am so glad we did.

Later, I realized that doctor suffered from his own fears and was in no position to help us. He had given up on solutions before he started, and he wanted us to do the same. But there was no damn way I was going to give up on Max in this lifetime. I walked away from the doctor's office with a feeling of disgust and being completely lost and hopeless. I had sought out expert medical advice but come away with more questions than answers. I didn't want my son's life to be over or to accept the fact that he would never reach his full potential and live out his true purpose. I feared I had failed Max, but I persevered.

My trust in so-called experts went down the drain. If the doctors couldn't help, then who would? Suddenly, I had an epiphany: it had to be us, as the parents. We would become self-educated about autism. We spend more time with our children than anyone else and should know them best. I had more than fifteen minutes to dedicate to my son's health, unlike most doctors with their patients. Once I returned home from the doctor's office, I had to do some soul-searching.

There were so many questions running through my mind. I didn't know diddly about autism, and the so-called experts had told me there was no hope for Max. How was I going to help him? The doctor was more educated than I was. He had a medical degree, and I didn't. Who was I to question what the doctor had told me? I remember those questions like it was yesterday. Who am I? I am his father and the very one who is supposed to protect him from people who utter nonsense advice.

At the end of the day, fathers do matter. In my mind, the FEAR was real and I was living it day in and day out. There was no escape and no waking up from this nightmare only to discover it's not real. My predicament was my life, and I was suffering. Later, I would learn that great suffering would lead to great learning, and I would see the world completely differently. First, though, I had to suffer.

If not for the suffering, I would not be sharing my story with you today and you would not be learning how to overcome your fears. I needed to find some meaning in my unavoidable suffering, a calling identified by famed psychiatrist Viktor Frankl. If I could just make some sense out of my experience, it would become more manageable. I chose to persist for my son, because his life is more important than mine. He may grow up to find a cure for some fatal disease, whereas I never will. This journey was bigger than me, and I believed that one day it would all make sense.

Today, I know I endured the tears, pain, heartbreak, sadness, disappointment, loneliness, guilt, and self-pity for my special little boy Max. Now, I want to pass on to you the knowledge that I have acquired from this journey. If I can help ease your heartaches, help keep your children safe, and somehow make your life a little better during the storms of this journey, then my hardship has been worth it. It all has meaning at this very moment. I know you are smart and willing to learn from my pain and suffering so that it might lessen what you have to go through.

FEAR BREEDS SCARCITY

I have met people who have lived their entire lives in fear. I've learned that fear breeds a sense of scarcity, because we focus so much on fear that we can't see anything else. For example, when Max was first diagnosed with autism, we treated him like a priceless piece of fine china. We were so fearful that something bad would happen to him or he would realize he was different from other children. We got fixated on all the "what ifs" that might happen. Life is going to happen regardless, and it doesn't care who has or doesn't have autism. What you think and do about it is what matters.

Looking back at our journey from Autism 2 Awesome, I often wonder how we made it through the tough times. I am talking about the day-in and day-out hardships, and I realized it was the blessings of God. Fear can take away our hopes and dreams, and it can eat away at our vision. Fear can have you thinking that you can't succeed because you've never heard of it being done before. When we allow fear to control us, we block the opportunities to become better than our best. And when we allow anything to stop us from being better than our best, then we are living a life of scarcity.

Scarcity includes believing there is no better version of yourself, which will cause you to fall into the trap of thinking there is no better version of your circumstances. There *are* better versions of you and better versions of your circumstances. You have to overcome your fears and allow yourself to discover the better version of you. I believe life is a learning process and we have the opportunities to become better people. We cannot do so when we allow fear to control our lives, and we cannot serve humanity living in fear. We all feel fear, but the people who push through it are the ones who go on to live the best version of their lives.

I lived a life of scarcity because of fear, and I don't want you to go through that any longer. Life is too short to live that way. Whatever you are going through, I want you to imagine the very worst of it. Really feel the sadness of it, and then get up and do something about it. Take a step forward through the fear. There is no scarcity in life, only the belief of it. Write down what you'll do today to stop living in scarcity. You can show kindness so that others know there is no scarcity of goodness in the world.

FOCUS ON THE SOLUTION

Here is what I did to overcome my fears and stop living a life of scarcity. First, I focused on the solution, which is exactly what I want you to do. Do something different than you have done in the past, and you will get different results.

I will share with you a little secret that I have learned along the way. It has been said what you think about, you bring about, or you may have read in your Bible that as a man thinketh in his heart, so is he. There is another way I have heard it said: wherever your thoughts are, that's where you are. I know when I was focused on the problems, I couldn't see a solution even if it was staring me right in my face. I couldn't even believe there was a solution. My mind was not open to the possibility of solutions, because I was fixated on the problem.

We cannot hold two thoughts in our mind simultaneously, no matter how hard we try. So when I focused on the problem, I got stressed, angry, frustrated, overwhelmed, sad, hopeless, and ready to give up. Life was in the process of beating me up and beating me down at the same time. I know it's tough not to give up and decide somebody else should handle your problem. It's tempting to say, "I am through, because this is too tough."

When I felt like giving up, I would see my little angel who was counting on me to find a way to help him reach his purpose. I had to find something else to think about—and fast. So I did. I started to focus on the solutions for my son and my family. Every day, I would challenge myself to see the world differently. What if this wasn't my greatest crisis but would become my greatest miracle if I could somehow wrap my mind around the right perspective? I needed to believe in myself even when nobody else believed in me.

When I was in elementary school, the teacher would read us "The Three Little Pigs." The simple children's story has a deeper meaning for me. It epitomizes facing a great crisis and having to come up with a solution. All three pigs came up with a solution of some kind, but the third one had a better solution that actually worked. All the pigs stayed focused on the solution and not the problem. See, I was one of those little pigs when I was told that my son had autism. I was running all around in a panic wondering what to do next. Autism was my Big Bad Wolf, and it was literally eating me alive. I needed to build a structure that would have a positive impact on my villain of autism.

I needed a house of bricks. That's right: I needed a rock-solid solution. But first, I had to go through trial and error. I could not build a house of bricks by focusing on my problem. I shifted my strategy and started to think about the solutions. I was amazed by the possibilities this kind of proactive thinking brought to my mind. It was like a light came on and there was nothing that wasn't possible. Solutions would take a lot of effort, but they were possible.

Solution-oriented thinking shifted the way I saw the world and myself. It decreased the amount of stress, anxiety, sadness, and anger that I was feeling. I realized that I had power over autism and choices about how to live. I had the power to help my son reach his full potential. Every day was a new day with a solid foundation that had been built the day before. I had the power to change my circumstances by first changing my thoughts. I had the power to change how I experienced the world.

What if Max's diagnosis of autism was an opportunity for me to become better than my best? This thought was exciting, and the possibilities were endless. As tough as I thought my situation was, I often thought about people who had a much tougher situation than me. This crisis in my life was about to teach me so much more about myself and what was really important to me. My fears of taking those first steps were slowing dissolving into a memory, and a new reality was being born.

At the beginning of my crisis, I thought the world had all the answers, but I discovered the answers were inside of me the entire time. Sure, there were days when my mind would dwell on the problems and not the solutions. But with practice, I would always focus back on the solution.

As Lao Tzu said, "The journey of a thousand miles begins with a single step."

So I began my thousand-mile journey. The first step of focusing on solutions instead of fear led me to the second step of overcoming it.

IGNORE THE FEARS OF OTHERS

The second step I took to overcome my fears was to ignore the fears of others.

When I first started to focus on solutions, people around me were not ready for this approach. They wanted to keep me in my fears so I could keep them company in their fears and misery. They didn't want to let me go, because they didn't want to be left alone with their worry. It's easy to get sucked back in to your old ways of thinking. When you decide to think differently and start focusing on solutions, you may lose one or two so-called friends you thought would stick by you regardless of your circumstances. Forward thinkers pay a price, but they also receive a greater reward.

If you lose people because you're focusing on solutions, maybe they weren't your true friends anyway. Just saying. My focus was Max, and I was not about to allow anyone else's thinking or fears stop me from helping him reach his full potential. Sometimes people can't process what you are going through; they are on the outside looking in. They can't comprehend the full scope of your challenges or appreciate the journey you're embarking upon. There is no reason to blame anyone for the way they process information. We all do it differently.

For me, I had to continue to focus inward, because I knew that's where the solutions were hidden. I had to unlock my potential so I could help my son with his potential. I was all in. I remember when I was working as a federal agent in St. Louis, Missouri, and I wanted to transfer to our Miami office to have a different experience. Almost everyone I spoke to had negative comments about Miami, but none of them had actually lived there.

At the time, I could not understand their motives for sharing their negativity with me. Later, I would come to realize no one can encourage you if they're afraid to conquer their own fears. I eventually moved to Miami, where I lived for two years. It was a great experience. Many times, your family and friends will think they have your best interest at heart, but they're focusing on their fears and not your strengths. The strength that you have inside of you is greater than anything. I had no idea how strong I was until it was time for me to fulfill my true purpose.

Helping Max reach his full potential was my true purpose at that moment. There were many negative things I had to ignore to be able to help him. I heard doctors know best, but the doctor didn't know my son as well as I did. I was told he'd be all right and not to worry about it. I was told maybe there was nothing

I could do, and that's just the way life is. Excuse me—I don't think so. Life is not just that way. I believe life is what you make of it.

These pieces of advice are all very logical if you are not willing to expand your way of thinking. I ignored them all and stayed on task. In the beginning, it was a lonely journey. Correction: it was a lonely journey, period. We felt we were on our own and that other people just didn't understand our plight. Now, I have people calling, emailing, and texting to ask if I can help them, and I'm always glad to share what I have learned.

During my research, I came across this quote by Bruce Lee:

> If you always put limits on everything you do, physical or anything else, it will spread into your work and into your life. There are no limits. There are only plateaus, and you must not stay there—you must go beyond them.

THERE ARE NO LIMITS

For me, Lee's quote describes the journey that Max and I shared. We didn't allow anyone to put limits on us. When you buy into the fears of others, you give them complete control over you and every decision you make. You allow them to limit you. During my greatest crisis, I refused to be limited by others and I refused to put limits on myself. I believe you don't know what you can do until you do it. If you want the best opportunity to become your better self, then you cannot allow yourself to be limited.

People often set limits on what they can do or will even try to do. There is so much more inside of you that goes untapped every day. Trust me: it would have been easy for me to look at where I was during my greatest crisis and put limits on myself. It would have been easy to say, "I can't do this," and give up. It would have been easy to buy into the fears of others, but doing so wasn't a solution for me.

I was continually in awe of Max's human spirit beaming from inside of him, just waiting to burst out and say, "Hello, world." No matter the outcome, I had to ignore the fears of others, because my son was counting on me. Many times, I felt tempted to put limits on my son and myself. I could have easily set low expectations after he was first diagnosed with autism, because I didn't know anything about the condition. Instead, I learned as much as I could about autism, my son, and myself. I could have limited myself and my son when the doctor told us to prepare him for a group home and concentrate on having other children. I didn't, though, and neither should you.

My family, friends, supporters, and I defied the odds and warnings of the doctor and chose to believe that something greater was possible. I could have easily set limits when my son first entered school, and the school initially refused to help, but I didn't. As his parents, we became his biggest advocates and used the resources available to help him get what was rightfully his, including a quality education. I could have easily set limits when he wouldn't sleep at night and I had to work early the next day. Instead, I developed techniques that would help him relax and sleep through most of the night.

There are no limits except the ones you put on yourself.

I never allowed any other person's fears to place limits on my hopes and dreams. I blocked out negative individuals, focused on the solution, and continued to seek every opportunity possible that would benefit my child. I knew the answers were waiting to be uncovered, even if the people around me could not see it. I could feel it, and I knew setting limits on his opportunities would not help him. I had to stay focused to get the best results.

When I moved to my first overseas assignment, my fears were at their all-time high. I had no idea what life was like outside of the United States, and neither did too many other people I knew. My first assignment was to Nicosia, Cyprus, a beautiful island in the Mediterranean Sea with wonderful people. Since it was my first foreign assignment, I had no clue what to expect. I remember first stepping into Cyprus and thinking how different everything was from the United States—of course, because it wasn't the United States. It was Cyprus, a totally different country with a totally different culture, cuisine, and music.

Cyprus was an excellent place to live. I would never have had this experience or other opportunities if I'd allowed my fears and the fears of others to limit me. I followed the same life strategy when it came to Max's health. If I'd allowed fear to limit me, then my son would never have experienced the life that he's lived.

He has lived in Ecuador for his final two years in high school as an honor student. He has played organized basketball and volleyball. He has traveled to different cities in Ecuador with the school and participated in community projects. Since this is a rather small community, he knows a lot of people and they know him. He has the opportunity to explore his surroundings and enjoy his freedom while making his own choices.

WHY ME?

Finally, I overcame my first-step fears by accepting the fact that I may never receive an answer to the question "Why me?"

For the life of me, I could not understand why our son had autism. Grappling with the reason was one of the biggest fears that kept me paralyzed. I would ask myself what we did wrong. Was this a punishment from God, and why did it have to happen to me? If I had other children, would they have autism? If I had continued to keep this kind of thinking in my mind, I never would have taken the first steps to overcome my fears. Instead, I would have continued to dwell in the unknown forever, and Max would have continued to suffer unnecessarily.

The unknown is the place of darkness where you can't see any solutions or way out. If you dwell in the place where you think life is bad, then life is bad—not because your child has autism but because you've chosen to limit yourself to a negative perspective.

In the beginning, I saw the very worst in my situation, and life returned the very worst to me. I was writing my own life movie, and it didn't have a happy ending. I was the movie star, director, and producer—and the victim. If I had been wise enough to be the observer, I would have realized I was my own worst enemy. If I could have seen myself from afar, I would have known much earlier that I was only looking at the problem and not focusing on the solution. I was petrified to let go of the problem for so many reasons.

I worried there were no answers—what if I couldn't help Max? The doctor had already told us to dramatically lower our expectations of our son's capabilities. I met other people who had children on the spectrum, and they were clinging to the hope of the doctors and what the doctors understood about autism. I had to learn to let go of everything if I wanted to help my son.

DON'T BE A CLINGER

What is a clinger, you ask? A clinger is a person who hangs on to something out of fear: old beliefs, relationships, fears, and old truths. It really doesn't matter what they cling to; they cling because they are clingers, and that's what clingers do. The sad part is they cling the most to what serves no beneficial purpose but actually holds them back—from self-development, happiness, personal growth, health, wealth, and reaching their full potential. What they cling to holds them back from being better than their best, and they pass the clinger mentality on to their child.

Are you a clinger?

I was a clinger. Like everyone else, I was so afraid to take a step and make a mistake. I had learned to cling because the doctors were supposed to know what to do, but they didn't have all the answers. At some point, I had to let go and smash against the rocks of life. It was hard mentally, physically, and spiritually.

At first, people tried to be understanding, but others thought I was just overreacting to a predicament I couldn't do anything about. I was sick and tired of the results that the doctors had produced, and I didn't like that I was allowing others to determine Max's future when they weren't even committed to helping him reach his full potential.

I stopped clinging and started realizing that life would only change when I stopped putting limits on myself. I just let go.

Once I let go, I no longer saw the world the same. I saw life from a different perspective and with different outcomes. I had learned to trust the process, and even doctors who were less than stellar were part of that process. Without having had a bad doctor, I never would have known what a good one looked like.

Today, I can say I am grateful to those doctors who asked me to give up on Max, because they made me more determined, stronger, and wiser. I learned to focus on the solution and not the question of why this happened to me. Sometimes crises will happen to you, but so do miracles. These days, I don't ask why—I ask what I am supposed to learn from the experience, which is a better question for me. It has helped shape who I am today. Nobody likes going through a crisis, but focusing on what I am supposed to learn keeps me on track and open to all possibilities.

I wish I had all the answers for you, but I don't. You have to take your own journey and discover who you are and what you are supposed to learn. What did I learn? I learned that life is beautiful, and no matter how tough you think you have it, someone else has it even tougher. Bad times don't last unless we allow them to. Love is real, and with it, you can overcome more than you think. The journey with Max inspired me to write of this book. I can't keep you from going through a crisis, but I can help you through it. I can share with you how I got through mine. That is my love to you. I can't stop your pain, but I hope I can show you what the other side of pain feels like—it's awesome.

DOS & DON'TS

Do take the first step because it's important.

Do focus on the solutions because they are the answer to your problem.

Do go beyond your plateaus because you have the potential to go higher.

Don't allow fear to control you.

Don't set limitations.

Don't be afraid to let go.

CHAPTER FOUR

IMAGINATION WITHOUT LIMITATIONS

"Imagination is everything. It is the preview of life's coming attractions."

—ALBERT EINSTEIN

After I graduated from college, I could not find a job, and I told my mom that I wanted to become a United States federal law enforcement special agent. At the time, I'd never met a federal agent. I didn't even know what you had to do to become one. I just wanted to be one so I could arrest criminals and keep the community safe. I wanted to make a difference and be of service to my community. I almost drove my mother crazy with the technique I used to reach my goal.

I used my imagination to develop a clear vision of what it would be like to become a federal agent. Because I didn't have any money, for a period of time, I moved back in with my parents. I would drive my mom around town so she could do her daily errands—to the bank, to the supermarket, and to visit her sisters.

Every time she left the car and went inside another building, I'd pretend I was doing a surveillance on her by talking into my imaginary walkie-talkie and giving a description of what she was wearing, how tall she was, and in which direction she was walking. Then, when she returned, I'd pretend to talk into my walkie-talkie again, saying she'd reentered the car. My mom would just look at me like I was crazy, and rightly so.

About two years after activating my imagination and working ten months as a federal corrections officer, I became a federal agent. This achievement was not an accident. I have activated my imagination plenty of times, and the results are all pretty much the same: astonishing!

CREATE A VISION

In the story above, I used my imagination to create a clear vision of what I wanted from life. I have used this strategy many times, and it has always resulted in awesome results. All of us have the opportunity to use our imagination to create whatever we desire.

The benefits of using your imagination are endless. My imagination allowed me to create a clear path for Max to reach his full potential and to live out his purpose. It also led to the development of life strategies for families raising children on the autism spectrum. That vision has added clarity to my purpose in life, which allows me to share my knowledge with others. I now have a greater impact on the world because of my imagination.

The downside of not using your imagination is wasting one of your most valuable resources for improving the quality of life for your child and yourself. Not using your imagination is detrimental, because your life will be filled with regret that you didn't give your all. The result is little progress.

HOW DO YOU IMAGINE YOUR LIFE?

How do you see yourself, and where do you see yourself? Have you ever asked yourself these questions? Why not? I asked them of myself many times when I wanted to accomplish something important to me as well as after our son had been diagnosed with autism. I was once asked if I thought Max would be all right, and without hesitation, I said yes. What else was I supposed to imagine—that he wouldn't be all right?

For me, imagining was natural and fun. See, I grew up in what you'd call poverty—not a lot of financial advantages. Correction: no financial advantages. Without these advantages, you have to use your imagination to get what you want since you don't have the money or other resources available to you. My siblings, cousins, friends, and I made up so many different games to play. You never heard us talk about how bored we were.

When the doctor said to give up on Max and focus on having other children, his mom and I were heartbroken. When we attempted to work with the school staff and they told us they didn't have the resources to educate our son, we were mortified. When we looked for resources and other professionals to help us, there weren't many to choose from. I was lost, but I had one thing that I could always rely on, and that was my imagination.

First, I imagined being my son and needing my father's help. What would I do? Then, I looked at my own childhood and asked what a better one would look like. I came up with how could I teach him in a fun, loving way without over-the-top expectations. I wanted to make every day a learning adventure for him. So I did.

MUSIC MAKES LEARNING FUN

My son hated to brush his teeth and would fight tooth and nail not to do so. I don't know if this was because he has autism or because he's a boy. Anyway, I wrote him a song called "Brush Your Teeth," and it went something like this:

Brush your teeth

Round and round

Brush your teeth up and down

Brushing your teeth is fun to do

Brushing your teeth is really cool…so brush your teeth

I would stand with him in front of the mirror and sing this silly song to him. While I was singing, I'd pick him up and move him back and forth in front of the mirror, all around and up and down while he brushed his teeth with no problems. From then on, he would ask me to pick him up so he could brush his teeth. This silly little song accomplished several goals. It stopped making bedtime a traumatic experience for him and me. It also allowed him to have healthy teeth and gums, and he had the opportunity to see his father act silly so that his little boy could be happy.

This short time in front of the mirror, singing and brushing our teeth, helped create a better father-and-son bond that has lasted to this very day. It also helped with his speech by practicing saying different words to the rhythm of a song.

When he was diagnosed with autism and later after he started school, the teachers told us that he didn't know the alphabet. I happily replied that he most certainly did. I told them to have Max sing the alphabet to them. Problem solved. Today, I have recorded about six or seven songs that I sang to him when he was a small child. I wrote a song about how to make friends, about why fathers do matter, and, my personal favorite since I wrote it, about why I'm so proud of him. When he would accomplish a small task that was a challenge for him, I'd make a big deal out of it. This song is upbeat and tells him how proud I am of him and everything that he can do. It starts out:

I'm so proud of you

Look at what you can do

I'm so proud of you

First you crawled, now you walk

Then you smiled, now you talk

I'm so proud of you

Look at what you can do

I'm so proud of you

Proud, proud, proud, PROUD

Then came your ABCs

And now you're learning how to read

I'm so proud of you

You're beaming all the time

Like a diamond with a shine

I'm so proud of you

You're very nice and really kind

Sharing with others all the time

I'm so proud of you

Look at what you can do

I'm so proud of you

Proud, proud, proud, PROUD

To this day, we sing the song as a family when one of us over-comes another challenge. It is the family theme song. I was amazed by how my son responded to the music that I created just for him. Now, I wanted to see how far we could go together and learn through music. So, I wrote a song about our journey from Autism 2 Awesome.

Now that I had music on my side, there was no stopping me. I was a madman who'd write a silly song about anything. Some were short, and some I recorded just for the memories. When I wrote the autism song, I imagined the two of us recording a video together. You can view this on my Autism 2 Awesome YouTube channel.

We all have doubts sometimes, and this autism crisis was my biggest one. No matter where you are in life and no matter what you are going through, you are awesome. You must believe that. It's great when someone else believes in you, but it's better when you believe in yourself. Your imagination is powerful.

LIFE'S COMING ATTRACTIONS

Remember what Albert Einstein said: "Imagination is everything. It is the preview of life's coming attractions." With music, I had a new tool in my hands, a new resource that I had never tapped into before. I was unstoppable. I have never been trained in any kind of music, and most of my friends will tell you that I can't sing, but it never stopped me from making music for my son.

The power of my imagination led me to music to help heal Max and me. Creating music for him was excellent therapy for both of us. It allowed my imagination to flow in all kinds of directions and develop programs to help Max reach his full potential. It offered an irreplaceable bonding time between us. I made the most of the moments regardless of how tired I was. I had a chance to be a part of something bigger than me: my son's future and the opportunities he deserved.

I had to be better than my best. Singing together helped with his language and boosted his self-esteem. Sharing music together was a fun time and eased stressful situations. I am sure it wasn't easy being a kid with special needs and having a high-strung father...seriously.

My imagination continued to expand with one idea after another. Each thought was the foundation for the next one. Each time I imagined something new, I'd imagine something else new. I reached the point where I started carrying a pen and paper with me because the ideas were coming so fast that I couldn't keep up. I was no longer looking for specific programs for Max; I was developing life-strategy programs for him. My programs were focused on helping him reach his best and fullest potential. Each one I created for him gave me the opportunity to engage with him and deepen the bond between us.

Then I had the idea of writing a children's book called *Daddy & Me* that I could read to him to help build his vocabulary. Also, I wanted him to experience seeing himself in a children's book. How cool would that be for him? Now, he has this story about him and his father forever. I wrote about some of the fun activities we shared together. The book helped to develop his attention span, which benefited him in school. It's been exciting for me to share it with other parents to read to their children, too.

The possibilities are endless when it comes to your imagination and what it can lead to. The rest of his brothers benefited from me reading the book to them as well. Once my imagination started to flow with ideas, so did his imagination. I could see what he responded to and why. I was beginning to understand my son and what worked and what didn't. The children's book has bright colors, laughter, and the two of us doing silly things together. But that wasn't the end of it—I wanted him to realize the full benefit of this experience. One day, I recorded him reading the book so we could play it back and listen to it. You can also listen to him reading it on my website. The experience was awesome and one I'll never forget. Now, I am working on a new book, *Mommy & Me*.

This journey has prepared me with the ability to teach others. We all have a great imagination, but children do in particular. It can be a rewarding experience to tap into their imagination as well.

ROLE-PLAY

Role-playing was significant in so many aspects in my life. I learned a lot from role-playing while participating sports and especially playing college football. As a federal law enforcement agent, role-playing was an instrumental part of my training throughout my entire career. The better your imagination is during role-playing, the greater impact it will have on whatever you're learning. You never know what life is going to throw your way.

During my good ole high school and college football days, we practiced all the time to make sure we were ready for game day. That's the way I look at the opportunity that I had with Max. Each day was training for him and for me, and hopefully whatever we practiced he would use to take care of himself one day. In sports, we would run and rerun practice plays until we could do them in our sleep. Many times, we would have other team members in different practice uniforms run the plays of the team we were going to play that week. Each game was recorded so that we could review it to see what we did right and where we could improve. I applied some of these same principles during my law enforcement career.

MAKING FRIENDS

I remember using the life strategy of role-playing when I was teaching Max how to make friends when playing on the playground. Most parents would like to see their children have friends, and it's a lonely feeling when you see that your child doesn't have any and has a difficult time making them.

I would demonstrate to Max how to go about making friends when he was on the playground with other children. The playground is usually where kids encounter each other the most, and a lot of social skills can be learned there. I'd get down on my knees so I was at eye level with him and pretend to be a small child playing. I'd create a scenario, and we'd role-play how to become friends.

As a first step, I only taught my son to say hello to the other child on the playground. After Max was comfortable saying hello, then the second thing I instructed him to say was his name. Third, I told him to ask the other child his name. Finally, he would ask the other child, "Would you like to play?"

All of this sounds good in theory, but then I started to notice the difference in how boys and girls played on the playground. I saw that young children, and especially boys, don't really play together at such a young age. They more or less follow each other around, kind of like "follow the leader" back in my day. After that, they move on to something else.

So, I instructed Max to do what the other kids were doing. We would practice this scenario of role-playing at home all the time. We'd also play "follow the leader," and I would allow him be the leader so we could work on him making decisions that were fun to him. This was a game changer when it came to using our imagination together and having fun doing it. When he had the opportunity to be the leader and I was following him, it boosted his confidence through the roof. Many times, our kids don't have the confidence that other children may have. But we can engage them in such a way that their self-esteem improves, and as they continue to develop, they will feel more comfortable being independent and asserting themselves in their careers.

PREPARING FOR SCHOOL

Sometimes, Max and I would play pretend school at home, which offered a fun way for me to get him excited about school and to prepare him for the real thing. I hoped going to actual school was going to be just as fun. I know school can be one of the biggest challenges for our children. It can be difficult for them to follow the teacher's instructions. The classroom temperature may be too hot or too cold. The lights in the classroom may be too bright for them. Our kids can become easily distracted by other children's behaviors in the classroom, which the teacher should address by assigning the best place for your child to sit during class.

In fact, Max does not like anyone being too close to him. If you are in his space, he starts to feel anxious and uncomfortable. We discussed some options with his teachers and found a suitable seating arrangement for him. The little things do make a big difference, especially to the child facing adversity. At the end of the day, it worked out for the entire class, because the less distracted Max is, the less of a distraction he is to the class.

While playing school at home, we would go over the alphabet, numbers, and whatever level of education he was learning at that time. We would also allow him to be the teacher to boost his confidence. As a result, he was able to start focusing for longer periods of time because he was more engaged with what we were doing.

For him, school became fun and interesting. Remember what I said earlier: if people are having fun, they can learn more easily, whether they have special needs or not. By playing school at home with him, I gave him the opportunity to preview the work the day before class, do the work in class, and review it again after class. We did our best to present the information to Max on multiple occasions in fun and interesting ways. This approach worked really well for us.

DON'T HOLD BACK

Research shows that drowning is one of the leading causes of death for children with autism when they wander away from their safe haven. I had already imagined the worst, and now I had to prepare him for the worst if there was no one else around to help him. I have to admit, with this one we caught a lucky break—a blessing.

Many kids on the spectrum are attracted to water, and Max was no different. I recognized my son's attraction to water was a strength. I used it to his advantage and mine. He was intrigued, so I started making up different games we could play in the water. I bought him little floats to put on his arms so he could see how it felt without me holding him. I remember him being in the water, totally submerged except for his head. He would maneuver his body so that he was spinning his body in the water. I was so proud of him. You probably figured it out that I made a BIG deal out of everything. I did—and you should, too. It is a great way to boost self-confidence.

I believe the smallest things can sometimes have the biggest impact.

One day while we were playing in the water, he stepped out of the pool and I asked him if he was finished swimming. He didn't say a word to me. I ask him the question again; still no response. He started to take off his arm floats, so I thought he must be finished swimming. Instead, he took them off and started stepping back into the pool. I said, "Wait, Daddy is coming—please wait for Daddy, baby." Too late—he had made up his little mind that this was the day he was going to conquer whatever he thought he had to conquer.

He jumped into the pool for the first time without his floats, and I was petrified. His mother shouted, "Let's see what he can do!" I asked her if she was crazy. I stood very close to him without grabbing him, and my little baby was doing his thang. I was awestruck. I thought, *WOW*. Maybe I'd been holding him back, and now he was showing and telling me, "Daddy, I can do it." Since that day, I have done my best not to hold him back. Sometimes it's hard, but I do my best. Whatever you do, don't hold your child back because you are afraid. If Max had ever wandered away from home or school, I was certain he would not have drowned.

Use your imagination and discover the endless possibilities of miracles.

BALLIN' 4 AUTISM: THE WORLD'S GREATEST INVENTION

Then it hit me. It had been staring me in the face the entire time. I had the world's greatest invention right in front of me, and I was about to use it to help Max grow to a whole different level in his achievements...Wait, wait, wait, you are saying you disagree with me. Let's take a look.

I want to share with you what I used to help Max develop life skills. It's the very same tool that helped me graduate from college. Are you ready to learn what it is? The world's greatest invention is the *ball*. Hold on before you fly off the handle. Just give me a minute to explain myself.

During my research, I came across the website YourTherapy Source.com and learned the entire brain activates when a child learns skills to handle a ball. In my rudimentary explanation, here is what happens. First, the brain will evaluate an object, and then it will identify it as a ball. The brain continues to analyze the differences between the ball and surrounding objects. After that, the brain finds the initial location of the ball and tracks the direction of travel. Then, the brain identifies the location of the ball, its timing, and where to catch it.

I believe the greatest lessons learned will come from life itself, and we learn the most when we experience a crisis. I also believe we learn best when having fun and engaging with that particular learning session. Every time we play a game involving a ball, we are having a different life experience and learning a lesson. In a game, we never know how the ball is going to bounce—and we never know what life is going to throw at us (no pun intended). Each scenario we face teaches us. In my opinion, games that use a ball prepare us for life by presenting us with different situations and helping us adapt to change.

When I was younger, I played all kinds of sports simply because I loved them. Unlike many parents today, mine never forced me to play anything or organized anything for me when it came to play. I never had a play date that I didn't organize myself. My parents didn't call some other parents and say, "I am dropping my child off at 3:00—can he play with your child for a couple of hours?" Who does that? Oh, we do. Why? Everything is so organized for our children that they no longer have to think for themselves. At a very young age, I organized all my playtime and I loved it. I played with other children simply because we wanted to have fun. That was it. Those times taught us more useful life skills than some students are getting in college.

DEVELOP LEADERS

Take a look at this: when I was younger and we played backyard sports, we had to pick teams. Doing so forced us to use our math skills to divide into the teams. We had two captains who were responsible for selecting the teams; they were usually the best and most respected players. They selected people they believed had a certain talent that would best benefit the team. Participating in this process introduced us to leadership, and we learned decision-making skills and analytical assessment.

Now, the kids selected for the teams were assigned to play different positions according to their skill level. The next time, they could try a different position, making them better players overall. This form of cooperation demonstrated trust in the players.

As I described above, the ball allowed us to use our communication skills and creativity while developing leadership skills. It also taught us that if we wanted to be part of a good team, we had to work hard. Being involved in a game that uses a ball developed our self-confidence, social skills, and situational awareness, in addition to promoting teamwork and broadening our networking abilities. Wow, until I said it out loud, I didn't know the ball could do so much. It can do even more for your child, because it is the world's greatest invention.

Playing with a ball develops the skillsets that companies look for when hiring new employees. In fact, corporations today sponsor outside work events for their employees to build morale and group cohesion. At these events, you will see coworkers playing games using the ball.

Many of our kids are not getting enough exercise, despite all the benefits that research has shown it to provide. When our children have the opportunity to participate in team sports on a regular basis, they will get enough exercise and also have a sense of belonging to something special and bigger than themselves.

Don't get wrapped up in worrying whether your child is "good enough." No one is good enough when they first start anything. When your child uses a ball to play against another child, they use their creativity, strength, hand-eye coordination, and balance. Plus, they're not sitting motionless in front of the TV. Participating in games using the ball constantly teaches about appropriate social behavior, how to make friends, and how to follow instructions. All these qualities make for a better entrepreneur, supervisor, CEO, teacher, father, and mother. I could go on all day, but you get my point. The world's greatest invention: the ball!

JUST START

When Max was very young, I started teaching him how to play basketball. He was terrible—and I do mean terrible—or maybe my high expectations made him appear that way (before I changed them). I was determined to improve his...everything.

I'd assist him with his dribbling. I'd stand behind him and put my hand over his hand, and we would dribble together and count each dribble, helping with his self-esteem and teaching him how to count early on.

Basketball also helped with science, physics, and reasoning, because he learned what would happen if he didn't bounce the ball hard enough or too hard. He learned that if the ball didn't have enough air, it wouldn't bounce—and you can't use a flat ball to play basketball, or any sport for that matter. Counting each dribble boosted his confidence and encouraged him to dribble even more the next time. He was eager to do so without me forcing him to do it. Since he didn't have any siblings and his social, behavioral, and communication skills were not fully developed at this time, I enrolled him in a recreational basketball league. At the time, the Paradise Valley Community Center in Phoenix, Arizona, was the best around, and I would put their programs up against others.

The first year Max played in the league, I was an assistant coach, and the five years after that, I was the head coach. I saw how my son started as this awkward kid with very few basketball skills. Then something happened: he became better at dribbling and pretty good at passing the basketball, and he even managed to score a few points in the game. I saw him become a kid just playing basketball and having fun. He was learning so much about life, but he thought he was only playing a game.

Sports have the power to change lives. Today, Max is an international traveler, an honor student, and a compassionate, respectful, well-mannered young man. He continues to play volleyball and basketball for his school here in Ecuador and has managed to make some friends while doing so. He is planning to attend college and is not afraid to try new things and give his all to activities he may not be so good at. He is AWESOME.

Most weekends, fans watch sports together and have a great time socializing and catching up on the good ole days. What a great stress reliever from the week. For just a moment we can share so much together by playing together. I believe many doctors, scientists, and inventors have taken a break from their hectic day to shoot some hoops, kick the ball, hit the ball, or throw the ball so they could relieve stress and clear their minds. The ball is the world's greatest invention, without a doubt.

The ball builds bonds between individuals or groups who share it. It can build great sports teams, or it can build great corporate teams. For me, it helped to build a great relationship with my son.

Remember the quote from Albert Einstein, and use your imagination to create your vision. Envision the life you want, and imagine life's coming attractions. As a reminder, music makes leaning fun and role-playing is a great way to teach our kids how to make friends. Just start with Ballin' 4 Autism—don't hold back, and begin developing our kids into leaders.

DOS & DON'TS

Do teach your child to swim, because it could save their life.

Do use the ball to develop life skills.

Do use your imagination to create your vision of a brighter future.

Don't forget to praise the small things.

Don't be embarrassed to sing and role-play.

Don't forget to make it fun!

CHAPTER FIVE

RESPONSIBILITY IS UP TO YOU

"The moment you take responsibility for everything in your life is the moment you can change anything in your life."

—HAL ELROD

After receiving an autism diagnosis for Max, I cried and then cried some more. I cried for Max, and I cried for myself. I didn't want this responsibility, and who was I to be given such a monumental task? I wanted to be a father by all means, but this was something different. There was no way out of it, and I was about to take the journey of my life. Someone had signed me up for something that I wasn't ready for. I didn't get the memo. Then I cried some more. *God, help me, please. Please give me a different responsibility that is just a little easier.* This future looked bad.

Recently, I came across this quote:

Your Attention Please: No one is coming to save you. This life of yours is 100% your responsibility.

The benefit of taking responsibility is that as you move through the process, you will develop life strategies to serve you and your family. Plus, it will provide you with a sense of control over your life. As you take responsibility for your own circumstances, your self-esteem will grow and so will your child's. The two of you will develop confidence in one another and learn to trust each other. When I took responsibility, Max and I developed a deeper connection.

The consequence of not taking responsibility is that your life and your child's life will be at someone else's mercy. This journey is your responsibility. I can't imagine allowing the doctor who told me to give up on Max being responsible for my son's quality of life. Failure to take responsibility means never having the opportunity to be better than your best. This is your journey, so own it.

YOU ARE RESPONSIBLE FOR YOUR CHILD—NO MATTER WHAT

As parents, I believe two of the greatest concerns we have for our special-needs children are who will care for them when we are no longer able and how to keep them safe. Many experts agree that early intervention is key to helping our children on the spectrum. I would add that as parents, we must also be consistent with the early intervention.

When I am developing life strategies, I like to keep the process simple and to the point, designing a realistic and accomplishable program. We decided early on that we were going to build a village to help Max develop and teach him how to care for himself. We started our early intervention techniques and remained consistent throughout his childhood. Although he is an adult today, we continue to coach him. I discovered through my personal life experiences that repetition played a major role in my success.

For example, I wanted to know what Max was learning at school so we could reinforce it at home, if we agreed with it. If we didn't agree with it, we could address it with school officials. We also frequently talked to the teachers at his schools to let them know what we were teaching at home so it could be reinforced at school. We wanted to repeat whatever he was being provided that assisted in his development, over and over. Every step of the way, we made it our responsibility to ensure that Max reached his full potential.

THE VILLAGE

As the African proverb says, "It takes a village to raise a child."

If we wanted to be certain that Max was cared for and safe long after we'd departed, then we had to take responsibility for putting those measures in place. We had to educate the villagers and develop a trust between us to minimize the possibility of something bad happening to our child. Who are the villagers? The people in Max's life on a regular basis. Here is how we did it.

First, I started with the adults in my family, because even after I accepted that Max was on the spectrum, many of my family members still didn't want to believe it. Nevertheless, I simply shared with them some of the life strategies we were implementing for him.

We informed our family that we had a specific eating plan for Max, because we'd discovered he was allergic to certain foods and other foods made him hyperactive. When he was hyperactive, he didn't have a peaceful sleep (and neither did we). They were skeptical at first, but after a while, they started asking if it was okay for him to eat this or that. Once he started to visit them, more and more my family observed his particular ways and had an opportunity or two to witness his autism meltdowns, which got them to jump on board pretty fast.

Secondly, we repeated the instructions above with the staff at Max's school. They were also slow to get on board, but with a little persistence and meetings with everyone responsible for Max's education, they eventually became great team members.

Finally, we got involved at the school. When it was Max's birthday, we took party hats, cupcakes, or whatever it took to have a great party. Most kids love a party, and his classmates would surround him asking, "Is that your mom and dad?" We developed such a good relationship with our village that a few teachers still attended his birthday party even when it wasn't at school. When others have the opportunity to meet you, get to know you, and see that you want the best for your child, I believe most will be willing to help.

Now, here is a life-strategy bonus that I simply love. If your child has siblings, cousins, or family friends of a similar age, you can ask the other children to help engage your child and encourage them to become buddies. You can explain in children's vocabulary that you child is shy, doesn't like loud noise, and doesn't like bright lights—or whatever you think are appropriate instructions. Children enjoy having some responsibility, so make good use of that impulse, because it changes when they become teenagers.

What did I do? Max didn't have siblings at the time, so I allowed him to mix it up with all his cousins and told the other children to come and get me if he needed me. Amazingly, when he was with the other children in his family, he never needed me. From time to time, I would peek my head in the room where they all gathered and ask how Max was doing. The other children would simply reply, "Fine."

I discovered he was learning through observation. He had the opportunity to observe the other children's behavior, and he responded appropriately. Yes, I am telling you first if you have never heard it before: kids learn from each other. As human beings, we all learn from our environment, whether it's good or bad. Most young children are at home, in daycare, or in school, so build your village and allow it to help develop your child.

I learned our family and school village was more than capable of making sure nothing happened to Max when we were not around. I actually think he enjoyed the break away from his parents. I know sometimes as parents we can be a little overbearing, or maybe it's just me.

FIND GOOD DOCTORS

Taking our son to a whole bunch of doctors and hoping they could help us turned out to be useless. I found I needed to take on several responsibilities real fast. As parents, it's our responsibility to ask the doctors how they can help us. Work with the ones who can help, and don't work with the others. It's our responsibility to find the best doctors for our children, not simply the most popular one. If we are to help our children reach their full potential, then we have to take responsibility for making that success possible.

Here are a few initial questions to ask the doctor:

- What is your background in helping children on the autism spectrum?
- What special training do you have related to autism?
- Do you have life-strategy plans relating to families with children on the spectrum?
- Are previous patients mainstreamed in school?
- Will you provide a nutritional plan for my child?
- What autism conferences have you attended within the last year or two?
- Do you work with other autism specialists?
- Are there other doctors or programs you recommend?
- Are any of you clients willing to share their experience with me?
- Do you have any success stories to share?

YOU ARE RESPONSIBLE FOR YOUR CHILD'S SAFETY
AUTISM AND SAFETY FACTS

The following facts were gathered from the National Autism Association's (NAA) website. For in-depth information and safety tips, please visit NAA's "Autism & Safety" site.

Drowning is among the leading causes of death for individuals with autism. You can google to find a list of YMCA locations that offer special-needs swimming lessons, and be sure that your child's last lesson is with clothes and shoes on.

WANDERING/ELOPEMENT*

- Roughly half of children (48 percent) with an autism spectrum disorder attempt to elope from a safe environment, a rate nearly four times higher than their unaffected siblings.
- Half of families with elopers report they had never received advice or guidance about elopement from a professional.

- Only 19 percent had received such support from a psychologist or mental-health professional.
- Only 14 percent had received guidance from their pediatrician or another physician.

Safety and security are some of parents' biggest concerns, and it seems the worry is magnified tenfold when a child is on the autism spectrum. I know it was a huge concern for me, and I have over twenty-eight years of federal law enforcement experience. I really had to use my imagination when I was developing a program to keep my son safe. Since becoming an autism advocate and teaching my techniques to others, I have learned some other methods from a few other people.

We had a major concern with Max's autism meltdowns. As you may be aware, these can occur anywhere. For us, they lasted from ten minutes to an hour or more. Minimizing them depends on the child and how well prepared you are. Seriously. When our son first started having these autism meltdowns, I had no freaking idea what was going on. They continued to happen over and over again. They weren't temper tantrums that lasted a minute or two, where you can reason with the kid at some point. I am talking about a full-blown meltdown, from zero to sixty miles per hour in four seconds. And I would think, *Are you kidding me?* I was really in crisis mode, because I wondered who acted this way. In reality, we all do at some point. I have seen adults

---

* Sources: Paul Law and Connie Anderson, "IAN Research Report: Elopement and Wandering," Interactive Autism Network, April 20, 2011, https://iancommunity. org/cs/ian_research_reports/ian_research_report_elopement; and Lori McIlwain and Connie Anderson, "Lethal Outcomes in Autism Spectrum Disorders (ASD) Elopement/Wandering," National Autism Association, January 20, 2012, https:// nationalautismassociation.org/wp-content/uploads/2012/01/Lethal-Outcomes-In-Autism-Spectrum-Disorders_2012.pdf.

behave worse than children, so I had to step back and come up with a new game plan.

I was quickly realizing my old parenting skills weren't working, and I had to develop a new strategy fast. I had another pressing problem to consider as well, because my son was nonverbal, and I couldn't ask him what he needed. He was speaking about fifty to 150 words at one point but had slowly regressed to only two to three words. Life really didn't seem fair to me at this point in my life…just saying.

While I was running around like a chicken with my head cut off, fate made me aware of a few strategies that worked really well for us. I remember one particular day was going less than perfect. A hurricane category 5 of an autism meltdown was in progress. I quickly put a cartoon DVD on the TV, and OMG, I saved the day for now, but I knew there were no witnesses except my son, who was nonverbal. He sat there and watched cartoons like nothing had happened.

Shortly thereafter, I replayed these events in my mind and wrote them down in my journal. I was attempting to identify what occurred right before Max had his meltdown. If I could identify the triggers, then maybe I could prevent a few of the incidents from happening. Just maybe. Also, his behavior was a huge safety concern. I recall one incident when Max was walking with his mother on the sidewalk in a shopping area. A motorcycle drove by and startled him, and he took off running across the parking lot.

We thank God that he wasn't hurt, but we learned from that day that he is not a fan of loud noises. The same applied to the movie theaters; we had to make sure that we were there before the movie started to play the previews. He would cover his ears and drop anything in his hands (so there went the movie snacks) when those previews came on. He would keep his ears covered until he had adjusted to the sound, and then he would still cover them periodically during the movie when he became too sensitive. Those observations became another entry in the journal. Hey, you never know when a family member may want to take him to see the latest movie and you'll have to explain to them: get there early, or you'll be sorry.

YOU ARE RESPONSIBLE FOR YOUR CHILD'S EDUCATION

I found out very quickly I was responsible for Max getting a quality education. If you don't know, then I will tell you that the educational system is broken right along with the medical system. School would present a challenge, but I was up for it even if I wasn't prepared for it.

For example, when my son first entered the school system, he had difficulty with his attention span and remaining seated during class, which was exacerbated by his very limited vocabulary. The school did not offer any solutions except to put him in a special-education class. I flat out told them, "This is not acceptable." I explained that he learned differently and needed more time to process the information given to him. The school didn't care to hear what I thought and didn't want what they perceived as a problem child. In kindergarten, the teachers were excellent as far as showing compassion to my son and us. When you're having a bad day, sometimes all you need is for someone to show you some compassion. It's always good to show kindness toward others.

I replicated the therapy so he could have more hours of it, and I made it intense. I was not about to wait until the state decided whether we qualified for an additional hour of therapy per week—give me a break. I could do it myself, and we did. The other problem was that the therapists weren't paid that well, so when a better opportunity came along for them, they were on to greener pastures. I can't blame them, though it made our lives more difficult.

Later, it was determined that our son would benefit from an Individualized Education Plan (IEP). We worked on his IEP as a team and all had to agree on what should be included in it. The IEP is a great tool to use for our special-needs children, because it makes tracking progress easier. The plan can be modified as needed. We were able to establish goals for our son and project when he should reach them. When he did, the team would establish new goals for him. Once we started working together as a team, it was a beautiful thing and helped him tremendously. The school district has resources that they should be providing to you, but you may have to do a little research to see what's offered.

We had regular meetings to discuss our son's education plan, behavior, attitude, and mood. If he is not happy, what's the use of a good education? I wanted him to be emotionally healthy, and over time, he was. A good IEP is a well-laid-out educational plan to help children reach their full potential. Every person officially responsible for your child's education should contribute to this IEP. You know you have a good teacher when they can comment on your child in a way that shows they want to help with his development and are truly vested in your child's best interest. I have worked with many teachers over the years and have been fortunate to work with some really good ones.

YOU ARE RESPONSIBLE FOR YOUR CHILD'S EMOTIONAL WELL-BEING

I had to be responsible for Max's emotional well-being. Every day, I thought about what our son was experiencing. He didn't have the vocabulary to express himself, so I had to be in tune with his emotions. In the beginning, I felt sorrow for him that his father wasn't a medical doctor and better equipped to help him. Then, I met a few of the medical doctors supposedly equipped to help him, and I knew he was better off with me as a father. No one could do what he needed other than his parents. I don't care how much education people have had; we knew our son, and we were learning about his needs every day.

Sometimes, Max would be sad and have autism meltdowns, and I just didn't understand why. I was responsible for his emotional well-being, and no one cared about our circumstances. If I didn't have insurance or the money to pay, my son did not receive that service or treatment. I was looking for anybody who could help us with our son. At that time, many doctors didn't offer any real solutions. Their first line of defense is always medication, and I wasn't on that page at all. You've got to do a little better, doctor.

We made the decision to heal our son and to take a look at our environment to see what possibly could have triggered autism in him and not others. We took responsibility and changed his environment completely. We changed his diet, the cleaning supplies in the house, the light bulbs, the toothpaste, and anything else we thought could cause him harm. We took precautions. From there, we started looking for good doctors who wanted to help Max, not push medication without knowing his history. It became our responsibility to find the best treatments, resources, doctors, and schools for him.

When we couldn't find what Max needed, we developed it at home to further his progress. It was my responsibility to make sure he received what he needed. Most experts agree early intervention is key to addressing autism. One of my earliest interventions was putting myself in my son's shoes and imagining what he would need from me as a father, including attention and consideration I may not have received as a child. I wanted to know what I could give him to continue his development. From our one-on-one time and conversations, I got to know Max and build a relationship with him. Those special times together taught me so much about being a better parent.

I recall riding by his school one day during summer break. The sign outside read, "Every Day Counts." It was talking about not missing school, but when I saw it, I realized that every day counts with my son. Every day counts with your child. I didn't have time to waste, and even though I didn't know exactly what to do, I was going to do something.

First and foremost, my early intervention technique was unconditional love for Max. I remember the love of my own mother and the difficult time she had educating me, and I wasn't on the spectrum. (At least I don't think I was.) Every day, I did my best to show him a little more love because I wanted him to know that in his home, he is safe and secure without any judgments. I didn't need a doctor's prescription, because this knowledge had been passed down from his grandmother (my mother), who taught it to his father (me), and I was passing it on to him.

Maybe one day he will pass it on to the rest of the world. Sometimes, this early intervention just meant hugs from me throughout the day, and no words were needed. It also included time together at the park going down the slide, or me pulling him in his little red wagon.

I remember leaving the park one beautiful afternoon after we had shared a magical morning there. I was pulling him in his little red wagon, and he was as happy as he could be. I just looked at him and smiled. I continued to pull him as we made our way to the car, and all of a sudden, the wagon became lighter. When I looked back, I saw he had fallen out. He was okay, so I didn't panic. What did surprise me was that he was still holding on to his ice cream cone. I thought to myself, "Where did he get the instinct from to protect that cone?" I knew he was much more capable than he was letting on, and even more than I realized. From that little lesson, I learned that I would use my instinct to help me navigate this mystery. He taught me so many lessons that I would have never gotten if not for him. There is a lesson and a blessing waiting for us every day.

SHARE THE KNOWLEDGE

I was just getting started with my imagination, and I was on a roll. Then, something hit me. I started thinking about various skillsets and how I could use them to help keep my son safe. I used a lot of role-playing to help him think about how to be safe, and we participated together in different scenarios. I would ask him what would he do in certain situations, and sometimes we would act them out. When I would give him the opportunity to be the leader, I could understand his thinking better.

As Margaret Meade said, "We should teach our kids how to think and not what to think." I wanted to teach my son how to think and continue to build upon that skill. In my nearly thirty years in law enforcement, I have had the opportunity to see many different scenarios and respond to them in training. These experiences prepared me for real-life situations, and I wanted to pass that knowledge on to Max.

I didn't stop there. I started sharing with parents how they could teach their children to be safer. My imagination continued, and I wanted to do more, so I developed a program for first responders on how to appropriately respond to situations involving children with special needs. Many police departments do not provide adequate training to their officers regarding responding to someone with autism. Officers are required to maintain a certain standard of training, and many of them are getting only the bare minimum.

The police are trained to go into a situation, take control, and use force if necessary. Many are never taught to de-escalate. I am speaking from experience; on numerous occasions, it was better for me to de-escalate the situation without using force. I have had opportunities to train law enforcement in the United States, as well as parents and school officials in the United States and abroad. Knowing what I know now, I realize I can have a greater impact on protecting our children through training parents, school officials, care providers, law enforcement, the judicial system, and all first responders. I believe autism awareness is great, but beyond awareness is autism training and education.

Finally, as a father, it was my responsibility to write down when I would spend time with Max. I wanted to make each day that I shared with him count. Most people will make doctor's appointments, hair appointments, and dentist appointments, and some people will mark their calendars for special meals and events so they don't forget and are on time. I made appointments with my son so he didn't think that I forgot him. I wanted Max to know that he was my most important appointment. So I wrote down when I was going to spend time with him and where we would spend our time together. I will have this memory forever, and so will he. He might be a little embarrassed by now as an adult.

DOS & DON'TS

Do take responsibility, because your child's future is your responsibility.

Do work with the school to develop an Individualized Education Plan.

Do remember: safety first!

Don't solely rely on others.

Don't forget emotional well-being for the child and the entire family.

Don't forget that dads are responsible, too. Get them involved.

CHAPTER SIX

SYSTEM OF ROUTINES

"You'll never change your life until you change something you do daily. The secret of your success is found in your daily routine."

—JOHN C. MAXWELL

As I reflect on my life, I now realize that everything I successfully accomplished started with a consistent system of routines. Along the way, these systems became a roadmap for me and many times resulted in success. They also served as a guide for the next goals that I wanted to accomplish in my life. I recall my early years in college when I struggled to keep up. I started to take copious notes for each class, and soon after class, I would rewrite my notes. Then before I went to bed, I would review my notes once more. I continued this routine all through my college years, and I received my graduate degree.

This chapter will explain how to build a system that is right for you and your family. You can learn to simplify your life and how to become successful. If you look at all the successful major companies, you will see that they have a system of routines—for example, UPS, FedEx, McDonald's, and Southwest, along with a host of other companies. If you want to be successful with your child, you need a system.

Not having a system puts you at a disadvantage. You will spend useless hours running in place and not making any progress. When we don't have a system and make little progress, it can lead to frustration and disappointment. Often this disappointment will lead to giving up on being better than your best. We need to continually make progress in order to be successful, and a system of routines can help us do just that.

One successful step can lead to another successful step, and so on. When you take that first successful step, you can reflect on your life to see where you have been successful and how you obtained that success. When I started a system with Max, it was my very first time attempting to establish a system of routines for someone diagnosed with autism. It would be one of my greatest challenges, because this person is our son. He trusts me to give him my best, and I trust what I have learned over the years of my life will somehow all come together to benefit him. Whenever we found a system of routines that worked for us, we implemented it in our lives.

I was scared to death. What if I was wrong? What if I made a mistake and made the situation worse? I am sure that I am not the only parent who has faced these questions and emotions, whether their child has special needs or not. I was no different from anyone else. I had been in tough situations before, but this time was different because it was our son and because I had no clue how to help someone who had been diagnosed with autism. Where would I even start? I really didn't know. I was shocked even to be told that Max had autism. I had to process what the diagnosis meant for him and his life. I wished the situation could be different for him and different for me. I had so much self-doubt as to what I could do to help my child.

I started to notice that Max had certain routines that he had to follow, or else. One day while he and I were driving home, I took a different route, and he started kicking the back of my seat and screaming. At first, I asked what was wrong. Then, I realized this was not the normal way that we usually drove home. I did my best to explain to him in a calm voice that I was still taking us home. I used my imagination to figure out the best way to calm him down quickly. Once our house was in sight, I pointed it out to him and he looked with such amazement. And yes, the meltdown was over.

So, how did I prevent incidents in the future? Good question. Any time I was going to deviate from Max's normal routine, I would prep him first. For instance, I would tell him, "Before we go home, I need to stop by the gas station and put some gas in the car." I would explain to him that we needed to stop by the store and pick up a few items, or I would say we were going home but in a different way. Prepping him allowed time for him to process what was going to happen next, so he wasn't surprised. The technique worked well for me.

FIRST, BELIEVE YOU CAN DO IT

My system of routines started with me believing that I could take steps to improve the quality of Max's life. I was not on the search for a cure, but I was searching for something better than what the medical community offered at that time. If I could find a small pebble of belief inside of myself that I could change someone else's life for the better, then maybe my life would be changed along the way. I have to believe. I have never tried to verbalize it before, but this belief was the first step and the cornerstone of success in my life.

I recall being asked once early on during those difficult days whether I thought Max would be okay. I responded yes. The person asked me how I knew, and I said I had to believe. What else am I to believe? Tell me this: how hard would you work to accomplish anything in your life if you didn't believe you'd succeed? You wouldn't work hard at all, because what would be the point? We had a long road ahead of us, and there was a lot of work to be done. Remember, I told you earlier in this book that I had no clue about autism, and here I was trying to make sense out of no sense. I was trying to unravel the mystery of what our child was going through, but I was completely lost. However, my belief in a force bigger than myself would guide me from one step to the next.

Whatever you want to accomplish today, start believing you can do it. You must believe. My mom was the first to encourage me to believe. When I was younger, I was not the best student…okay, I was failing school badly. My mom would regularly plant little seeds in my subconscious about how I could do it if I just put my mind to it. She'd have talks with me about listening to my teachers and doing my best in class. She provided me with a lot of support. Her guidance when I was younger played a vital role in my professional and personal success. I saw her take a similar approach with my siblings, and we all have gone on to live productive lives and have children of our own.

She believed in us long before we started to believe in ourselves. I wanted to give that same type of environment to Max. No matter what, I wanted him to know that I believed in him. So how did I do it? Every day, I did my best to show him that I believed he could succeed. I planted small seeds in his head about how smart and special he was, telling him he had certain talents that others didn't have. I also talked with him about how he would have to work harder in other areas, because others have talents that he doesn't have. I know you already understand that there were a lot of frustrating days, and trying to put together a routine was going to take a lot of patience.

I understand that life can be difficult at times, and my life was extremely difficult after I learned Max was diagnosed with autism. Every day, we have the opportunity to plant seeds in our mind that can help us outlast the bad times. We have the opportunity to plant positive seeds into the minds of our children, too. I believe if we water these seeds with love, support, self-esteem, laughter, and positivity, there are no limits.

Proverbs 22:6 says, "Train up a child in the way he should go; even when he is old he will not depart from it."

At first, it may seem like the seed will never grow and produce something of value. But first you must plant it and give it the best opportunity to grow from a system of support.

ANTICIPATE THE NEEDS OF YOUR CHILD

The second thing I did was to understand and anticipate Max's needs based on our past experiences together, figuring out how I could address those needs on a daily basis. I realized that I was not going to prevent many of the difficult times that he and I would experience. However, I could minimize the length of his unpleasant experiences—and mine, too.

When I started his system of routines, it was simple trial and error. When I discovered something he liked, I'd write it down in my journal and make sure to use it again next time. One of the first techniques I used when he would not sleep, or he was very hyper and we wanted him to calm down, was to take his little foot in my hands and give him a foot massage. I found he really loved this activity, and it would calm him down and get him ready to sleep. It became part of our system of routines that continued into his teenage years. The massage not only calmed him down but also played a huge role in our bonding time, contributing to our relationship to this very day.

He grew to understand that his father would give him a foot massage at bedtime. He looked forward to it, and so did I. Max had trouble sleeping, and I anticipated that if he didn't sleep well, neither would I. The foot massage would end the routine of the night, and he knew afterward it was time to go to bed and sleep.

Before the foot massage, he would have his warm bath with all of his favorite toys in the bathtub. He would play with his toys, and I would make up silly learning games to help increase his speech and language skills. I tried any fun game I could come up with while he was taking his bath. While he was in the bathtub, he enjoyed the water and was really, really calm, and we like calm. There was no anxiety about being in the water; in fact, it was the opposite—he loved it. So I turned that time into a learning session and a chance to bond with Dad.

After he was finished with his bath, it was time to brush his teeth. He hated to brush his teeth, and looking back, maybe he didn't like the way the toothbrush or the toothpaste felt in his mouth. I'm sorry I didn't realize it then. I got creative by writing the silly "Brush Your Teeth" song to sing to him while he looked at himself in the mirror. Picking him up and making a big production out of the task got him to smile and laugh, turning it from a stressful time into a positive one. I anticipated that this system of routines would give me the most opportunity to be successful and both of us to have a peaceful night's rest.

We discovered some routines the hard way. Once, I remember putting Max in his bed for an afternoon nap so he and his parents could relax. We lived in a ranch-style home, and it was a gorgeous day outside. We decided to leave the window up so he could have fresh air. Moments later, I heard a noise coming from his room and decided to investigate. This little boy had kicked the screen from the window and was standing outside of the house. It scared the bejesus out of us. Fortunately, our backyard was fenced in and there was a second security gate that protected him from the swimming pool. His mother was totally freaked out (I was a little bit, too).

So we started using monitors for his room, and when we heard him stirring around, we always got up to see what was going on. We also kept the window closed and locked in his room, and he got fresh air when we all went outside together. Using one of the skills that I developed in my law enforcement career, I started detailing every incident and making notes on what could be done to prevent such occurrences in the future.

You can develop routines for tasks you frequently do with your child, such as going to the grocery store. It sounds simple enough, but I highly recommend that you hold your child's hand when you are walking out of the store. If they're small, place them in the shopping cart. If they're hesitant, then make a game out of it. To prevent accidents, I also recommend after leaving the store that you secure your child in the car seat before loading groceries into the car. That way, if someone tries to take you against your will, you can jump in your car, lock the doors, and drive away, with the child already safe in the vehicle. You can always buy more groceries.

Always have your keys in your hand before you leave the store so you don't have to fumble around looking for them. When it comes to safety, always be aware of your surroundings. Keep it simple.

At home, I like to take my child out of the car first before unloading the groceries and get him situated inside where he's familiar with the surroundings and has his own routine.

DISCOVER THE BEST SYSTEM OF ROUTINES FOR *YOU*

Like many parents, we discovered early on that Max liked things in a certain way. Even before we had received a diagnosis, I recall a day when he had taken all of his small toy cars and lined them up in a perfectly straight line on the floor. Then, he just lay on the floor staring at them. I think he would have stayed there most of the day if we had allowed him to. In his young mind, he already had a system for dealing with his possessions. Everything had to be a certain way.

He didn't want certain foods touching each other on his plate, and while riding in the car on the way home, he only wanted to take a certain route. He only wanted to sleep in a certain bed, and he wanted certain toys when he was taking a bath. All of these routines worked well for him personally, but I needed them to work for him to be a success in society. I had to understand what system of routines would work best for him. There was a lot of trial and error, and we both learned along the way. He definitely taught me that he was not going to give up his own established systems. He was comfortable with the way his life was.

During my high school and college football years, all of the practices were on a system. In practice, we would go from one drill to the next and repeat our plays over and over so often that we could do them in our sleep if we were asked to. The experience introduced me to my very first good studying model. From this technique, I would learn the importance of seeing the material I needed to learn multiple times. The duration wasn't as important as the frequency of seeing the material.

Similarly, we would teach Max what he needed to learn using frequency. Our desired goal was to show him what we wanted him to learn multiple times, using short intervals. For example, when we taught him to tie his shoes, we would make a game out of it so that he could learn one step at a time. We would practice that one step multiple times throughout the day. When he was ready, we moved on to the next step of tying his shoe. The goal was to make him successful at the task he was attempting to complete.

In football, game day was our big test to see if we'd learned what we had been practicing, just like reviewing your school-work during the week to prepare for the test on Friday. I hope you understand where I am going with this. We learned these skills using a ball…the world's greatest invention. (I bet I made you smile.) My coach would always say, "We are going to get it right if we have to stay here until the cows come home." If you are from Alabama, you know the cows don't come home until the sun goes down. These systems of routine would later help me in the classroom, my career, and my entire life. Systems have worked for so many people, companies, and especially the military.

One of the early systems that we started was to read to Max. Since he was only using limited vocabulary, it helped a lot. Reading together gave us the opportunity to build a closer bond and allowed us to help him increase his vocabulary and especially his sight words. These are some of the most commonly used words that are usually not phonetic, so you have to know them by sight (hence the name "sight words"). Today, he is an excellent reader.

As Max got older, he continued to use a system of routines that assisted him with being successful. He has developed a clear vision of what he would like to accomplish, and he does something every day that leads him toward completing his tasks. Because we started when he was younger, he developed self-esteem over the years that convinced him he could succeed on his own. This system of routines that we started turned into a life-changing set of habits for him.

Because of those early years, Max can now anticipate his own needs and plan accordingly. He has truly discovered a system of routines that works best for him. He has his own way of doing things, and I am completely okay with that. He has gone from barely speaking two words, not focusing in class, and having total meltdowns to learning how to develop routines that make him successful. I am so proud of him.

DOS & DON'TS

Do believe that you can succeed at helping your child, because you can.

Do anticipate the needs of your child.

Do have a system of routines that work best for you.

Don't worry about the trials and errors, because you can learn from them.

Don't forget the benefits of a system of routines.

Don't forget to keep those doors and windows closed and locked!

CHAPTER SEVEN

TEAMWORK: YOU ARE THE CAPTAIN

"Alone we can do so little; together we can do so much."

—HELEN KELLER

Why should you be the team captain? The better question is why shouldn't you be the team captain? You don't need to know everything about autism to be the team leader, but you do need to be dedicated, committed, and open to the possibilities of your purpose. Now, what is your purpose? That's for you to decide. For us, our purpose was to help our son to be happy and healthy and to improve the quality of his life. Today, we've succeeded, and he's striving to reach his full potential. He has accomplished so many goals along the way. Soon, he will decide his own purpose and how to go about achieving it.

This chapter will help you understand the role of the captain. It's not about being a dictator but rather doing what's right. As a captain, you cannot allow your ego to get in the way of your child's future. You must hold the team together, despite your hardship—and there will be hardship. You must be able to see the bigger picture, which is making circumstances better for your child.

If you don't understand the importance of teamwork, then you will never be successful. You'll miss out on others' input to help your situation. Your child will suffer, and there will be little progress. No matter how smart you are, you can be smarter as a team. Have you ever heard the old saying that two heads are better than one? Every person who has experienced some success in life has benefited from others' support, mentorship, and coaching. We all need someone just to be there for us.

During my senior year in high school, I was named co-captain of the football team. In my youth, I did my best to be a good leader by example and a good teammate. I worked hard every day to be my very best. Later in life, my approach paid off when I realized I am the captain of my life. You are the captain of your life as well.

Being the captain of my family meant being better than my best to help Max reach his full and best potential. I had to be better than I had ever been before if I was to be successful. Of course, there were many obstacles to overcome, but these only made me stronger. I saw them as being like a hard workout, just as lifting weights offers resistance that helps build muscles. Sure, there is some discomfort from the training, but after a day or two, that discomfort goes away and your body feels better. I always stretch before and after my workout, which further helps my flexibility.

To me, being the captain of your destiny is similar because there will be resistance in life, and we must become stronger in order to overcome it. All of us will face challenges that stretch us, but that stretch will help us build character, confidence, and self-esteem. As Steve Maraboli says, "A life unchallenged is a life unchanged." The world is constantly changing around all of us, and we must challenge ourselves to adapt to change while breathing through the resistance and learning how to stretch with life.

At times, I felt like giving up, and at some point you may feel like giving up also—but don't. When I felt like giving up the most, I didn't realize how close I was to a breakthrough. I want you to remember: when you feel like giving up the most, a breakthrough is about to happen. At the moment of feeling defeated, you are close to witnessing a miracle. Keep going because you are the captain. As the captain, you inspire others to continue despite the difficulties. When they see you, they see hope, strength, and a better tomorrow. You are the captain.

Not so long ago, the doctor told us to give up on our son, prepare him for a group home, and focus on having other children. As you know, Max is not preparing to live in a group home but instead preparing for college. He has taken advanced courses that I'd never heard of. Life has given us the opportunity to work with talented people and create the best team possible for Max. A good team will improve the health and the quality of life for your child, but how can we recognize talented people?

FIND TALENTED PEOPLE

When you are the team captain of your child's future, how do you go about finding talented people who can have a positive impact on your family? I mean people who are committed to what they are doing. When our son was first diagnosed with autism, we faced a serious problem of finding and retaining talented people with appropriate training. They were in short supply. If you were fortunate enough to meet such a person, they were already booked working for multiple families. If by some miracle you had such a person working for you, they didn't stay around long, because there were so many other opportunities for better pay. At least, that was my family's reality.

To build a talented team, we cast a wide net. We started our search in the usual places, asking the school about individuals who might be looking for part-time work and contacting all the local resource centers that work with special-needs children.

In addition, we sought out family members who could get training to assist us. We were particular and didn't have family members who lived close to us. We lived in Arizona, and after Max was diagnosed with autism, we completed all the required paperwork and applied for assistance through the state programs. We received a certain number of hours for trained individuals to come into our home and work with Max. The hours were very limited, and if a person was really good, they weren't with the agency for very long. Then, we'd have to start all over with someone new. At the time, we didn't know much about autism, so we would watch how they worked with Max and replicate what we saw the therapist doing. The approach worked well, and we learned a lot. Then, we noticed how we could modify the program and customize it for the needs of our son. We would ask teachers for referrals of anyone looking to work part-time and train them.

At one point, we had a couple of college students majoring in education working with Max. During that time, we were going to a lot of different doctors, conferences, and workshops, and we would ask everybody if there was anyone they could recommend we work with.

I suggest you cast a wide net and be open. Some of the people you come across may seem unlikely to help you, but they may be a diamond in the rough. It's perfectly normal to proceed with caution before allowing someone in your home to work with your child. You can always ask for letters of recommendation. Also, use the internet to find out additional information about them. Do your homework before letting anybody into your home. Trust your gut instinct. I prefer meeting people in person so I can get a feel for them, and if that feeling ain't right, then you can't work with my child. This rule applies to the highly educated and also to the not-so-highly educated. It has worked for us in our personal lives for the past fifteen years.

In fact, I remember a gentleman who was scheduled to work in home with Max. I asked him a few questions regarding his background, and he seemed enthusiastic about his work, which I appreciated. I shadowed him and Max during his first visit. At the end of the session, I asked him a few other questions regarding his background, and he seemed reluctant to answer them. He had a great personality, but his reluctance to be forthcoming led me to decide he would not work with our child.

TEAMWORK IS BETTER WHEN THE WHOLE TEAM WORKS TOGETHER

Now that you have this talented team assembled, how do you go about getting them to work together? If you have selected the right people, there shouldn't be any major issues, but there will be some growing pains.

First, stay focused on improving the quality of life for your child and the whole family. One of the ways that our team stayed focused on Max's quality of life was by using a journal. We went through multiple volumes by the time we were done. All the team members (therapists) who came to our home contributed to the journal, and we asked the teachers to send home notes, which we also added to the journal. Our journal offered a detailed account as to what occurred each day, week, and month.

As we read the detailed accounts from each day, we could understand what he had experienced. We did this for years, and the journal also served as a measurement of his continued academic success. When we visited the doctor, we had our trusted journal that we could refer to and better explain any changes we'd noticed in his eating habits and sleeping patterns, as well as any decrease in his verbal language. The journal tracked the number of hours that he had slept and whether he exhibited any food allergies.

Good communication is key when it comes to successfully accomplishing your purpose, and the journals allowed us to effectively and clearly communicate with our team. The team exists to improve the quality of life of the child and family, so stay focused. Identify and clearly define the roles of each team member.

My family learned that it is not only the person with autism having a tough time; the entire family is going through a crisis. You can decrease stress by getting the entire family to exercise, such as by taking walks in the park or playing basketball together. We had this big old trampoline that he loved to bounce on. If you don't have room for a big one, they sell the smaller ones that can go inside your house or garage. I have already mentioned swimming and the importance of teaching our children how to swim and be safe. The entire family can experience all of these exercises together and make them really fun. I tried to keep Max moving as much as possible, because for me, just sitting around doesn't keep the brain active enough. I taught him how to ride a bike, and we got him involved in martial arts. Stay active. Keep them moving. Keep that brain working.

RESPECT THE VALUE THAT OTHERS BRING

Some of the best team captains I can think of have always valued what others had to offer. When my family and I were going through our darkest period, we looked to the medical experts for their advice. But there are so many different components to helping someone with autism. There is also a common-sense approach, which you may not get from the medical field. The point is that a person can only teach you what they know, and no one knows everything. So, we valued the educators on our team because they brought the academic component to the table. Plus, many of the teachers we encountered were very experienced as our son entered the higher grades. Based on Max's social behavior and academic achievement, the teachers were able to tell us how he was developing compared to typically developing children. Even if we didn't initially agree with their assessment, we valued the experience they brought to the table. We listened to them and were open to hearing their explanation so we could process the reasoning behind their thinking. This approach led to better communication and cooperation on both sides.

We valued the therapists who came to our home at the time to work with our son. Their training allowed them to bring a different component to Max's program. We always asked questions to better understand why some therapists worked one way and others took a different approach. Either way, I made it a point to learn from them. I was open to finding the best way to help Max. There are a lot of people willing to help you, but you have to give them the opportunity. I learned something from every person who was involved with helping my Max reach his full potential. When people feel that you value and appreciate their experience, it means a lot to them, and usually they will give their all in helping you.

One of the best ways I have found to value others' experience is to ask them how we should go about implementing what they've suggested. Give them the opportunity to own it and further help them see they are an integral part of the team. I believe a good team captain helps people feel valued. As Maya Angelou said, "People will forget what you said, people will forget what you did, but people will never forget how you made them feel."

STICK TOGETHER

As a young man in college, I tried out for the football team and eventually earned a football scholarship. During one of our seasons, we made it to the playoffs and only needed to win two more games to become national champions. Most of the team became homesick, because of what we thought we were missing. Football practice started in early August, before the other students reported to school. We would practice three times a day, five days a week, for a few weeks, and then the schedule would change to twice a day. When school started, we only practiced once a day for five days a week and played our games on Saturdays. As the season progressed, Christmas break was upon us. The student body was on vacation for about three weeks, but our football team had made it to the playoffs, and we remained on campus.

As a team, we started to lose focus about winning the championship. We started to think more about being home and enjoying

Christmas break just like the rest of the student body. We wondered what all the work was for and whether it was even worth it. Then, we lost in the second round of the playoffs and got our wish to be home for Christmas like everyone else. If we could have been just a little bit more mentally tough and drawn from each other's strength, we could have won the championship. Instead, we indulged in each other's weakness, and we lost and went home.

Personally, one of the greatest lessons that I have learned from playing sports all of my life is not to feed off of others' negativity. Everybody can't do what you can do when it comes to your child, and everyone will not be as committed and dedicated as you are, either. Remember, you are the captain. Act like a captain and lead the way. The following year our football team found ourselves in the same predicament as the one before. We were right back in the playoffs, but this year was different, because before the very first practice, the team captains called a meeting to talk about the prior season. That day we all made a commitment to dedicate ourselves to the purpose of winning the National Championship, no matter what obstacles got in our way.

We made a commitment to one another to have the best attitude for each other and not to defeat ourselves just because we were a little tired, cold, hot, sweaty, bruised, hurt, or homesick during the holiday season. We declared this was our time to make history, no matter what. That year we won and secured our place in the school's history forever.

The moral of the story: a good captain helps the team stay focused. A good captain can reenergize the team when everyone is tired and can continually remind everyone of their purpose.

It's time to be the captain of your team and reimagine the typical stories about families of children with autism.

NEVER LET SCHOOLING INTERFERE WITH EDUCATION

Novelist Grant Allen, a contemporary of Mark Twain, said, "I have never let my schooling interfere with my education."

I've mentioned that Max had a difficult time when he started school. A good captain is creative and understands that learning goes beyond the walls of a building.

At first, the school administration and teachers were not friendly or understanding of the challenges we were facing as a family. There was no compassion or empathy for a family who had a child recently diagnosed with autism. I used my experience from sports to build a team to educate Max. We cultivated and developed a team out of individuals who weren't used to that kind of collaboration.

In the beginning, the school officials wanted to take the path of least resistance, but they quickly discovered we were not going to allow that to happen. We offered to coach the teachers on the best ways to work with Max. At first they resisted, because they were not open to the possibility that our son could learn. Apparently, nobody wanted to put the work in for our child who was going through a crisis. But I made sure that I put the work in at the school and outside of the school. At that time and at that particular school, many of the teachers weren't trained in educating children with special needs. Remember earlier when I suggested that you start a journal? Well, we already had one going, and we used it to coach the teachers and keep the other team members well informed. Our journal informed his teachers if he had a bad night of sleep and if he was currently constipated. I don't know about you, but I ain't learning sh** if I'm constipated (no pun intended). It is hard enough to learn when you have a neurological challenge, without the added discomfort. Yes, we kept notes on everything.

We consulted with the teachers on how he learned best. We advised that whenever they could put the lesson in a song and include movement with him, they would see better results. We made notes about how often we did different activities with him. We always made it fun, intense, and in short bursts. We would do different activities all day, but they'd last for ten minutes. For example, we would turn the music up and dance with Max until he broke a sweat. He loved it. This activity allowed us to continue to build the family bond. Furthermore, we would play different kinds of music and see which one he liked the best. We would discuss which music he liked and why. The dancing was great exercise for him, and it helped with working on his coordination. The dancing also helped him to burn off some energy and sometimes led to a better night's sleep. These repeated activities built his self-esteem and encouraged him to have fun exploring life.

After dancing, we'd eat something healthy, and then it was time for a book with Daddy. We made books come alive. We had a true adventure with our reading time. By acting out the book and bringing it to life, he had a richer experience with learning. We read all kinds of books involving appropriate social behavior, and we would talk about why it was good to be kind to other people. We shared everything that worked at home with the school and our entire team. While wrestling with Max, I noticed that he liked the deep pressure of being hugged or playing "tickle time" with me.

We noted where he was sitting in the classroom and who was sitting next to him, because we realized all of these particulars could affect his mood, his attitude, and eventually his learning. We educated ourselves about our son, and he was the only person who could teach us about him. You will not get this kind of education from a doctor. We coached the school on all of these details, and we explained how learning to address his needs would benefit the whole school. Whatever the teachers learned from us had the potential to empower and prepare them for children with autism who entered the school system after Max.

Remember: you are the captain of the team that works together. Always communicate the common goals of the team. Search high and low for talented people, and when you find them, stick together. Remind the team how valuable they are, and let them know how much you appreciate their dedication. Remember to always respect others and what they bring to the table. I believe we can accomplish so much more with the help of others.

DOS & DON'TS

Do be the captain and lead the team, because you are the best person to do it.

Do build a talented team, because we all need help to be successful.

Do value other people's feelings.

Don't delegate your child's future to someone else.

Don't allow obstacles to let you lose focus.

Don't allow schooling to interfere with your child's education.

CHAPTER EIGHT

RESILIENCE

"She stood in the storm, and when the wind did not blow her way, she adjusted her sails."

—ELIZABETH EDWARDS

When I think of resilience, I think of being able to overcome a crisis and using what I have learned to improve my family's life and the lives of others. My greatest crisis was hearing that Max has autism. I felt as though my world had ended, but it was only a new beginning. In this chapter, I want to share with you that our family experienced the fear of rejection, and as parents we felt as though we didn't have much to offer to our son. But with each day we grew stronger and realized the value we could add to our child's life.

You shouldn't sell yourself short, because you are valuable. At the end of the day, your situation is not as bad as you think. Life is about the visions we create for ourselves.

I want to help you, too, discover that you have resilience. In fact, you would not be reading this book if you didn't have what it takes to bounce back from your crisis and improve the quality of your child's life. What you have done thus far has the possibility to inspire others to be better than their best.

Don't miss the opportunity to find just how much resilience you have already shown along with the dedication and commitment to reaching your miracle. Each day when you get up and do something to improve the quality of your child's life, you take a giant leap in your thousand-mile journey. I want you to know what you are truly capable of.

I needed to be able to bounce back from my crisis. Personally, I had to be able to logically assess the situation and then resolve it, accept it for what it was, learn from it, and move on. I always did my best later to be thankful for the lesson, even though I didn't enjoy it. I believe we need a sense of gratitude, knowing that we are still here and have the opportunity to start new chapters in our lives.

We choose how to write the next chapters of our lives and not our circumstances. Sometimes, we may need to forgive others and ourselves. We are not perfect, and we don't have to be. I am convinced that it is healthy to forgive yourself. We will not always get it right—no one does. After forgiving myself for thinking that I didn't know enough about autism to help Max, I was able move forward. I was able to progress. Prior to this forgiveness, I was stuck in disbelief and unable to logically piece the puzzle together. Forgiveness gave me a new mindset, which paved the way for a more positive conversation to take place inside my head. My conversation changed from self-pity to wondering how I could learn more about autism and help improve the quality of life for Max.

Whatever you are going through right now and whatever you

are feeling is part of the journey. It will be hard and it will hurt, but in the end, it will be helpful. We're guaranteed to be blown around during our lifetime, so we must learn to be resilient to stay on course.

THE FEAR OF REJECTION

Sometimes what seems like rejection actually turns out to be opportunity. As author Steve Maraboli said, "Every time I thought I was being rejected from something good, I was actually being redirected to something better."

Once Max was diagnosed with autism, my negative thoughts allowed my fears to control my life. I didn't want him to know that he was different from all the other children, and I didn't want society to judge and hurt our fragile child. As parents, we asked ourselves, do we keep him hidden away from the world to protect him from all the ugliness that may come his way, or do we choose how we live despite our circumstances? Do we teach our son to run and hide when life starts to get a little tough? I DON'T THINK SO.

In my life, I was accustomed to dealing with discrimination, unfair treatment, and people shunning and attempting to discourage me from being better than my best. I learned at an early age that life will not always be fair, but life also taught me to use what I've learned to grow and help others grow. I recall those days of being frozen in time and not wanting to get out of bed and deal with my life. But I had to, because there were people counting on me. I can vividly remember the heartache of dealing with the schools that wanted nothing to do with Max. I can remember the stares from other people looking at us and judging us instead of offering some compassion.

We lived in fear most of those early days. There was the fear of our son being victimized and taken advantage of when he was away from us. There was the fear that he might never speak, be able to make friends, go to parties, and one day graduate from high school. We also feared he would wander away from home or school and be injured or killed. Like many other parents, we worry ourselves sick about our children.

It's one thing for something to happen to me personally, because I know I will eventually bounce back from the situation. It is completely different when something happens to my child. Still, I have found that life experiences are the best teachers, and they have taught me to be resilient.

From those experiences, I knew I had to face my difficult challenges head on. There was no easy route and no way to avoid the pain. I made it a point not to hide Max from the world. I was prepared to do my very best to prepare him for what he would encounter during his lifetime. It was no secret: he was different from typical children, and the world would treat him differently as well.

I choose to approach this situation the same way that I have approached other challenges in my life. I began by remembering my purpose to Max, which included giving him the opportunity to be happy and healthy and to reach his full potential. I took a logical approach. Using logic is not always easy, because you're dealing with a beloved child and the many emotions involved. I get it, but we must continue to push forward. I wanted to develop his skillset so he would be able to care for himself with limited assistance from others.

THERE IS ALWAYS HOPE

A small thread of hope allowed me to remain optimistic about his future, gave me strength to fully recover from any setbacks, and motivated me to continue on. My resiliency started from being hopeful about Max's future and the wonderful possibilities that waited for him. In simple terms, I held on to hope for his success in my mind and used a common-sense, logical approach to consistently bounce back. Once again, I wrote in my journal about any setbacks that I had and possible ways to correct them. I was always searching for the best way to make progress. Once you start writing about what you could do, your mindset and perspective will shift. All kinds of possibilities will present themselves, and the resilience will grow.

I would remind Max of the circumstances that I thought he would encounter in life. I would explain to him how to deal with difficult situations and tell him to focus on how he could better himself by learning a positive lesson. I believe that holding on to negative feelings about yourself or others is self-defeating. We talked about ways of developing emotional growth from our everyday experiences. The process of developing life strategies for him was fifteen years of constant conversations and coaching. Often when the negative voices started to speak to me, my emotions would run wild, and I would become frantic about what might happen to my child in this world.

After regaining my composure, I would refocus on hope regarding Max's accomplishing awesome things in his life. I saw the positivity he brought to every person he encountered. From him having the opportunity to meet others, he unconsciously expanded their consciences as well. Some realized how fortunate they were not to have the struggles of raising a child with autism. Others realized how gifted these children are and wondered about their potential. I often wondered about Max's potential as well. He thinks so differently than I do and is so compassionate. Since we decided not to hide him away from the world but rather to face the public and challenges head on, Max has been blessed by the experiences he has gained. I believe others who have met him have been blessed as well. Remain hopeful, and focus on your purpose to help your child and you. Doing so helped me become even more resilient over the last fifteen years.

DON'T SELL YOURSELF SHORT

Since we didn't know much about autism, we searched high and low for the best experts to help us. Fortunately for us, Max's mother was a voracious reader, an excellent researcher, and an overall badass when it came to understanding and processing large quantities of technical information quickly. In a few years' time, she knew more about autism than the doctors we were seeing. Once we realized that some of these experts did not have Max's best interests in mind, we changed our strategy. We became self-reliant and the most knowledgeable about his health. Max's mother would attend many different autism and health and wellness conferences while I stayed home with him. Once she returned home, she'd share with me what she'd learned. During those early years, there were many different approaches being espoused about autism, and none of them appealed to us.

She tackled the nutrition and medical aspect, and I tackled the early life strategies, education, physical fitness, and safety. Between the two of us, we concentrated on the development of his emotional intelligence. We wanted to make certain that Max was developing into an emotionally well-adjusted child. We paid close attention to his attitude toward school and his classmates. We'd ask the staff whether he was happy at school and felt a sense of belonging to the group. Along the way, we kept an open mind, and his mother frequently attended autism conferences that we could afford. There was always informative advice, and we continued to learn each step of the way.

We stopped having negative self-talk and focused on internal conversations more in line with accomplishing our vision. We all have a voice inside of us at some point in time telling us what we can't do. We have to overcome it and allow the positive, encouraging, self-confident talk to take over. We will never be as resilient as we can be if we don't change the way we talk to ourselves. I realized the following:

- There is no other person with me more than I am with myself.
- There is no other person talking to me more than I talk to myself.
- There is no other person who can influence me more than myself.

Through resilience, I learned that I had a lot to offer to Max—I just didn't know it at first, because I heard the word "autism" and fear automatically kicked in. In fact, I could now teach my son to be resilient. We could all use more resilience, whether we are autistic or not.

There are certain things that Max can only get from me, and there are certain things that only you can give your child. I am confident that you have so much to offer to your child, your community, and the world. Don't sell yourself short. Take an inventory of what you are good at, and use it for good. If you think that well-put-together people have it all figured out, then think again. We all struggle with something at some point, and the struggle can be a good thing. Don't be afraid of what you don't know, because all of us don't know something. Allow yourself to be stretched and uncomfortable—if you're not uncomfortable, then you're not learning.

I recall early on when I was developing Special Intervention Training Techniques (SITT) for Max and a lot of people didn't understand what I was talking about. Upon further examination, I realized that evidence-based research was already there to support what I was doing for my child. You can google the benefits of exercise and physical fitness. Earlier in this book, I provided information on how the brain works when you are catching a ball, and all throughout the book, I've shared with you what hard work does for us. Don't ever sell yourself short because someone doubts what you are doing. You may be the next person with the big breakthrough to help our children live their best life possible. Remember: if you sell yourself short, then you are selling your child's life short.

IT'S NOT AS BAD AS YOU THINK

It's a bad feeling when you don't know the way, and trust me, I have been there many times. But it's not as bad as you think when you know there is a way. Like any life crisis, raising a child with special needs is a very tough situation to adjust to and overcome. As I look back on our journey, I can say it was difficult and there were some really bad days. There were times when we didn't have the money to see a certain doctor we thought Max would benefit from. There were many times we could not afford to hire additional support for him. Often, it was just the three of us, and we got little sleep. I worked crazy hours back in those days, but my day didn't end when I got home, because my son was so glad to see me. When I got home, it was his time to be with Daddy, and I am grateful I made the extra effort to be with him during those early years.

At the time of his diagnosis, I felt as though I was living in a nightmare that would never end—the constant meltdowns, sleep deprivation, lack of understanding from others, depletion of life savings, and sense that all our hopes and dreams were quickly fading. All of the above sounds bad, and it is if you focus on it. I told you earlier that meltdowns can be minimized. Learn to sleep when your child is sleeping. Some people will understand, and more will follow. Finances can be replaced, and your hopes and dreams depend on you.

We did our very best not to get caught up living the dreams of society and other people. We allowed ourselves to have realistic hopes and dreams for Max. For us, each day was a new beginning building on what we had experienced and learned the day before. As we defined who we were and understood our purpose, the challenges didn't seem so bad. Eventually, we could see the big picture and ignore all the inconsequential distractions.

We made our own little world that benefited our family and created a healthy environment that supported our purpose and our vision. Soon, our world became normal to us, and in our world, anything was possible. We were able to see small miracles every day, and life seemed okay. We found joy in helping Max and seeing his awesome progress. Eventually, we started sharing our knowledge with others, and for me, there is nothing more compassionate than being of service to your fellow man. Our mind is the most powerful tool we have, and we have the power to create the future and world that we want to see. Remain hopeful.

DOS & DON'TS

Do know that you have the ability to bounce back.

Do trust who you are and who you are becoming.

Do find your purpose.

Don't be overcome by fear.

Don't stop being hopeful.

Don't sell your child's future short.

CHAPTER NINE

EXPOSURE AND EXPERIENCES

"If there is no struggle, there is no progress."

—FREDERICK DOUGLASS

Recently, Max participated in Model United Nations in Quito, Ecuador (a one-hour flight from Guayaquil), with his school, the InterAmerican Academy. While there, he and his classmates had mock debates regarding global issues with students from different schools. He attended several formal events, where he had to dress in business attire. The entire conference took place in Spanish, but he was allowed to speak in English to argue his points of view during the debate. This was his senior year studying at the school.

In this chapter, I will share with you the importance of exposure and experiences in improving your child's quality of life. Some of the topics I'll address are communication, unexpected surprises, experiences to grow from, and good values. I learned just as much from these topics as Max did.

There are no limits when it comes to exposing our children to different experiences. With each experience, our children walk away with a newfound sense of wonder that surrounds each of us. They also gain a sense of self-confidence that continues to grow.

If you fail to grasp the importance of exposure and experience, you risk hindering your child's growth and development. Your child may never experience the sense of wonder and curiosity that inspires so many of us. You don't want to deprive your child of the opportunity to use his gift of imagination to change the world.

COMMUNICATION

Help your child to find their voice. The ability to communicate is so important, whether you are on the spectrum or not. I had to find a way to help Max find his voice. During our challenges, he had regressed to about two words. I wanted him to be able to communicate with the rest of the world. Children can express themselves through speech, art, music, dance, technology, and many other means. We exposed Max to various experiences to see what resonated with him when it came to communication. At the time, we didn't know which form he'd prefer, but we tried different ones. Now, he is excellent at public speaking and art. He has learned to express himself through drawing, which he loves to do.

After Max returned from Quito, I asked him how Model United Nations went and whether would he like to do it again. He responded without attempting to be funny, but it was funny to me. He said, "Dad, I am a senior this year, and I won't be attending this school next year, so I can't be a part of it." I just laughed. I then asked if he had the opportunity to be a part of it again whether he would do it, and he said yes. I asked him if the trip was fun and exciting. He told me that it was kind of boring, but he learned a lot. He added that he spoke about technology and economics while representing the country of Argentina. He admitted that he learned how to articulate his arguments to defend his point of view. He said he learned how to use facts to make his argument stronger and more influential.

Max was excited about the overall experience and having the opportunity to participate. If he had not been exposed earlier in his life to drama, playing organized sports, and interacting with the public, I don't think he would have had the foundation needed to successfully participate in Model United Nations. After graduating, he decided to take a year off to work and do some traveling in Europe before starting college in Arizona. He knows exactly what he would like to major in. He is conversational in Spanish, which is his second language. He has a social group that he engages with, and he has played basketball since he was eight or nine years old.

UNEXPECTED SURPRISES

I'd like to share an exposure and experience story with you. The athletic director at Max's high school emailed me and said that I needed to pick a most valuable player, most improved player, and most potential player since I was the head coach of the basketball team. I looked at the players I had on my team and what they all had contributed to the season. I picked the MVP with no issues, and the team voted on its captain with no issues. Now, it was up to me to decide who had improved the most. I had one person in mind, and then after careful review of my son's contributions, I had two people for consideration. I was hesitant about selecting Max, because I didn't want to seem biased toward my son or unfair to the other kids. On the other hand, if he had improved the most, I didn't want to be unfair to him and not select him.

Before I made my decision, I spoke to the athletic director about other matters, and he shared with me that he had been to all the games except one or two. He said Max had a great season. I was in total agreement with him. Max and one of his teammates shared the recognition of most improved players. If Max had not been exposed to playing basketball at a young age, he would have never been in a position to be recognized for his hard work and talent in basketball. He would never have learned how to work hard even when you are not the most talented on the team. He would never have built camaraderie with teammates sharing a common goal of working together to win something important to each of them or known what it feels like to try to reach his full potential. I have seen his dedication and hard work transcends sports and carries over to his educational studies and everything else he shows an interest in. He would have never had this exposure and experience if we had been embarrassed about his condition.

For me, I would have never seen how this little boy would face adversity and go forward to accomplish so much in such a short time. I get teary eyed when I think about the obstacles he has faced and overcome. I know being exposed to different situations and circumstances afforded him a different experience, which has given him a solid platform to make better decisions in life. Over the years, these exposures and experiences have given his brain a reference point to relate to. He could not have expanded his perspective if we'd sheltered him. I am confident that he is able to identify solutions to his challenges and implement them.

EXPERIENCES TO GROW FROM

One of the first things they ask you when you interview for a new job is "Tell me about your experience." The potential employer is asking this for a reason: they want to know what have you done, what are you looking to do, and what can you do for them. They want to know what value are you bringing to the company. If you are not adding any value, why should they hire you? If you want to give your children an opportunity to excel and to learn how to think, then give them exposure to different experiences and watch how they grow and reach their full potential. I have seen children who have everything planned out for them by their parents, teachers, and other caregivers. Later in life, this micromanagement can hinder some of these children from making decisions for themselves. They have to live with the consequences of not being able to think for themselves.

Typically, I have found these kinds of kids are afraid of failing. I don't think most parents understand that failing is where the learning takes place and that you can never truly fail if you never give up. Max has been exposed to a lot of different experiences, and I am still surprised by the things that he doesn't know. However, when I was his age, I didn't know half of the things that he is capable of comprehending right now. Every day, I see this young man who in so many ways is still my little boy. The exposure and the different experiences have helped shape his forward thinking today.

Max took several Advanced Placement (AP) math and English classes during his junior and senior years at his international school. Many people don't realize what it takes to reach your full potential, and I really wanted to give this gift to Max. I always impressed upon him that there is no giving up, no quitting and going home. My efforts were to teach him that you find a way to accomplish what you want out of life, because your life is your responsibility. He's a young man now. I love him and am proud of him for the way he has accepted the challenges and responsibilities that have come his way.

There is no way he would have adapted to the enormous changes of living in a different country and going to school abroad if not for the exposure and experiences that he had early in his life. Many of us want to protect our special-needs children from all the negativity surrounding the challenges of having autism. As Max's parents, we had to have a heart-to-heart talk with one another about how we wanted to raise our son and what we wanted for him in life. We knew we wanted him to be healthy, happy, and able to think for himself. We wanted him to reach his full potential.

One summer when he was fourteen or fifteen years old, we enrolled him in a summer drama program. My hope was that the class would help him to be more outgoing, become a little more talkative, make new friends, and see life from a different perspective. He has always taken his studying seriously, and I wanted to show him that you can learn something new while having fun. OMG, when I saw him perform his three different sketches at the end of the program, I was blown away. I could not believe this was my child. He was completely into his character and engaged with the other characters, even when they veered from the intended script. I told him that day he should go into acting, whereas before he attended the summer program, I never would have suggested that he consider acting as a career. I was amazed by his ability to perform. The entire family saw the video of his performance, and everyone was equally impressed. They were pleasantly surprised by his flexibility in portraying different people in each scene. He was the star of the show, which was an amazing exposure and experience for him and gave me a different insight into my son.

Another time, I was at the school and we had just finished with basketball practice. One of the teachers asked me if Max had told me about being interviewed by the students from the journalism department. I said no. She explained that during the outdoor school, the senior class went to do community work for a less financially fortunate school. She said Max and the students were interviewed about their experiences helping others. She told me that out of all the interviews, his was the most thoughtful and thought-provoking and that all his classmates agreed. If not for the early intervention exposure and experiences, he might never have wanted to live abroad, participate in drama class, take dance lessons, or try out for the varsity volleyball team. The way I see it, our kids have compassion and kindness that others should see. Our children have so much of value to offer, and the world really needs it at this time.

GOOD VALUES

I compare exposure and experiences to building a house. When you build a house, you need to start with a strong foundation. With a weak one, the entire structure is in jeopardy of crumbling under the slightest pressure. My parents provided me with a solid foundation of good morals. I knew right from wrong, and I respected people because my mother didn't play with regard to her children disrespecting anybody. She instilled the foundation of good character in my siblings and me at an early age, and I am grateful.

My parents also instilled in us the value of hard work. They taught us if we wanted something out of life, we had to put the work in to get it. I passed these values on to Max starting from early childhood. When his teachers told me he was so polite and kind, it made me feel good to know he practiced these values. I always let him know that I love him and am proud of him. He is capable of learning; he just learns in a different way. I never wanted to deny him the exposure to different experiences that would allow him to grow and develop into a caring and kind human being.

With each experience came a valuable lesson about life. For example, when he would get upset, I'd ask him about the cause. He'd share the reason with me. I'd ask him how being upset felt, and he'd tell me. Eventually, after a series of questions, we'd reach the conclusion that he doesn't like being upset. Then, through a series of questions, we'd see how we could look at the situation differently to have a better outcome.

I had my share of embarrassing moments, but I survived, and so did Max. Each exposure gave him a different experience to refer to the next time a similar situation occurred. I was determined to give him a solid foundation. It all started at home, without the need for a doctor's prescription. I was able to use what I had learned from my exposure and different experiences as a guide to assist Max to reach his full potential.

My career took me to different parts of the United States and then to places like Cyprus, Africa, Ecuador, Spain, the United Kingdom, France, Italy, Israel, Jordan, Greece, and many others. Those exposures and experiences opened my mind to other possibilities and opportunities. I have been fortunate enough to be able to pass this perspective on to Max. He has had the advantage of seeing other parts of the world through his own eyes and having his own experiences. I have witnessed these experiences transform him from thinking strictly about academics to being a global thinker and a more compassionate person. He has had the opportunity to visit less fortunate neighborhoods in Ecuador and share knowledge with others. He was also able to use some elbow grease to help paint a school, clean it up, and feel good about making a difference in someone else's life. I believe we must give our children the opportunity to think for themselves when they are young if we want them to be able to think for themselves when they are older.

LET THEM FLY FREE

I'll never forget the moment I found out Max had autism. I would never wish the experience on any parent. I was devastated. I was prepared to do whatever it took to protect Max from all the pain I thought he would have to endure. I was about to be that helicopter parent who always hovers around to protect my child from feeling the slightest bit of discomfort.

I wanted him to grow up strong, be able to think for himself, and show compassion to others. I was about to deny him his rights of passage because I was allowing my fears to take control. I wanted him to one day be able to fly off to his own destiny. I have met countless parents who hinder their children's ability to fly.

When I was a young man in my early twenties, I enjoyed lifting weights and having a hard workout. The slogan back then was "no pain, no gain." You had to work those muscles in order for them to grow. I had to find my own inner strength to allow Max to struggle and help us both grow. I knew his struggles would make him stronger, wiser, and definitely more appreciative of his accomplishments. Once he was able to overcome a few challenges, he would then be able to overcome a few more. His confidence would grow, and he would continue to find his own inner strength in life to achieve even more. Based on my own personal experience, I had developed a map that could guide him to success. He could modify this map however he chose, because it was only a guide. I taught him there are many ways to have success in life and he just had to discover what success meant to him.

As parents, we started our early intervention with our son immediately after we received the diagnosis. Our goal was to help him reach his full potential without limiting his vision. This is what I mean: some people live their potential based on the beliefs of their parents, whether or not they have special needs. They live for someone else and not for themselves. For us, one of the first strategies was to teach Max to take care of himself and have fun doing it.

We started with teaching him to pick up his toys. Then, we progressed to teaching him to make his bed. Back in ancient times, when I went off to college, I was very surprised by how many people didn't make their beds or put their belongings away. I believe learning these routines early in life will benefit you later in life. As you get older, putting away your toys becomes putting away your clothes. I heard a speaker say when you make your bed, it gives you a sense of accomplishment at having completed a task and is a great way to start your day. You can build upon the feeling for the rest of your life. When I talk about developing a system, it can be as simple as making your bed every morning and cleaning your room to start the day. Small accomplishments have the opportunity to grow into additional success. When our children are successful within their own environment, they are unafraid to leave the nest and fly toward new adventures.

SOCIAL EVENTS

There weren't many birthday parties or other social events for Max to attend at first. The few times he did attend birthday parties, his behavior didn't meet the hosts' standards, and we were never invited back again. As a father, I had to find ways to get him exposure to different experiences that he could learn from. I know firsthand how the right exposure can change a person's life. When Max was in kindergarten, he was a loner and really didn't have any friends. He was not equipped to advance to the first grade at the end of the year. He remained in kindergarten for an additional year, which was a good decision on our part as parents. It gave him additional exposure to being around other kids and starting to learn the basics. As I reflect back, I'm actually elated that he had this experience. The teachers at this particular school were kind and compassionate, and for that I am forever grateful.

As his behavior became more socially acceptable, he began to make friends and got invited to more birthday parties. He would also have his own parties and invite his friends to our home. These experiences eventually taught him from a young age to bounce back from the disappointment of not always being invited to a party. Now as a young adult, it is not such a devastating experience when he is not invited to a social event.

FUN AND NOT-SO-FUN EXPOSURE

One of Max's first exposures was not a great experience. I can laugh about it now, but it wasn't so funny at the time. I signed him up for the soccer team while we lived in Phoenix, Arizona. If you have ever been to Phoenix, you know the temperature can get hot enough for you to scramble eggs on the sidewalk. Let's just say my son didn't fare too well in the Arizona heat. During practice, I would offer him water on a regular basis, but it didn't help. I would learn later that he prefers cold weather. After the soccer season, we started basketball training inside the gym, out of the sun. Lesson learned.

The next exposure and experience was swimming. At first, I kept him in floats and monitored his every move. Once he tried floating on his own, though, I saw he knew how to tilt his head back in the water and maneuver his body in such a way that he could go around in circles. He was having the time of his life, without any stress or worry. I was amazed when I saw him and wondered how he learned this skill, because it wasn't from me. We shared a lot of moments in the pool, and I had to trust his instincts, though I stayed close by and observed just in case. He has been swimming ever since, and the experience was a good one.

I discovered early on that if I limited his exposure and experiences, I was not allowing him to grow and develop into a person capable of reaching his full potential. I allowed him to fall and fail, because doing so offers some of the best exposures and experiences in the world. Society would have us to believe that everyone gets a trophy for participation. That attitude may be well and good in a controlled environment, but real life doesn't work that way. Our son will face some serious issues, and it is up to me to prepare him and teach him how to get what he wants from his life. I know when it comes to having honesty and integrity, he will not cheat himself or anyone else. I am proud of all he has learned and feel confident he can take care of himself.

Each day is an opportunity to learn and an opportunity to teach. Make each day count to show children how to take care of themselves. Just take a look around at the real-life, everyday experiences and help your child to become engaged. If you are baking in the kitchen, allow your child to help you and make a game out of it. When your child wakes up, make a game out of making your bed, washing your face, and brushing your teeth. Our children love routines, and we can use those habits to teach them to be successful. All the habits that we teach them at home are transferable to school, the workforce, and adult life. Being disciplined is a good habit if you want to accomplish any kind of goal and live your full potential.

THE ROAD OF CRISIS LEADS TO THE FREEWAY OF MIRACLES

Max's autism diagnosis has taught me more about life than anything else. My story likely has similarities to yours, whether your journey involves autism or any other crisis right now—whether it is the health of your child, career disappointments, or your own health problems. It doesn't matter what it is, because you and I have the ability to survive and thrive. We have to learn to hang on a little while longer.

I felt every bump of this crisis road, and I thought the ride would never end. But as I continued to hang on for dear life, I discovered the journey can be shaky at times but every bump gave me more appreciation of life. This road humbled me and gave me the opportunity to reflect. I knew somewhere a family was having a much more difficult time than I was. I made a promise to myself that when I got to the other side of this crisis and could bask in my miracle, I would help others realize their miracles also. What is the point of me gaining all this knowledge if I can't do some good with it to help others?

I found my purpose in my greatest crisis of all. When I needed help the most, I felt the call to help others. I didn't enjoy the suffering, so I wanted to do well and serve humanity based on my experiences. We can all benefit from such sharing. Along the way, there were outstanding people in my corner, and they are still here today. They encouraged me not to give up and when they saw the progress Max had made, they encouraged me to help others as well. I love helping people, and I enjoy working with kids to teach them new skills. That is my life's purpose, which is why I have dedicated my entire adult life to serving my community in law enforcement as a federal agent. I have had an opportunity to impact others I've met along the way, and they've made an impact on my life as well. It has been a win-win situation for everybody.

I was promoting Autism 2 Awesome Life Strategies at an event, and a family came over to me. The mother started talking to me about her son. I listened to her carefully, and she started to cry. I asked her why, and she said she didn't know if she was doing the right thing for him and wanted him to be okay. Her husband and other two children were standing behind her while she spoke to me. As she continued to cry, I asked her and her husband if it was okay if I gave her a hug. They both agreed, and then I asked her a few questions and for permission to speak with her son who was diagnosed on the spectrum.

When I spoke to this little boy, he blew me away with his intelligence and his vocabulary. I asked him a few questions and told the parents he was really smart. I asked if they'd had him tested as a gifted child. I told her, "Whatever you are doing, keep doing it, because you are doing a wonderful job with him." I also told her that sometimes boys are just boys; they want to try to push the limits. Don't get caught up in labels. Then, I shared my story with her about how the doctors told us to give up on our son and focus on having other kids—and about Max's achievements over the years.

We shared tears and laughter. Days like that one reaffirm my purpose to continue being of service to others. That family had a powerful impact on me, and I hope I was able to encourage them that their crisis would become their miracle also. Most of us are just trying to do our best with what we know. If you are coming from love, then you are on the path to doing the right thing. I always do my best to keep an open mind and continue learning. Along the way, I didn't get it right a lot of times, but I didn't use my mistakes as an excuse to give up and stop striving to be better than my best. The love you have for your child is one of the greatest exposures and experiences they will ever have. Keep it up, because it goes a long way on the road of a crisis that leads you to the freeway of miracles.

DOS & DON'TS

Do expose your children to different experiences, because they can make a big difference.

Do teach your children communication skills.

Do build your child's social network, because it is a valuable tool.

Don't think the bad experiences are not good exposure.

Don't keep your child from flying, because they deserve to soar.

Don't doubt yourself.

CHAPTER TEN

SPECIAL INTERVENTION TRAINING TECHNIQUES (SITT)

"Ignorance is always afraid of change."

—JAWAHARLAL NEHRU

As you are well aware, experts do not know the cause autism. However, they do agree that early intense intervention is a key factor in helping children who are on the spectrum. Most of the early interventions that you will find focus on the child who has been diagnosed. In fact, once a child receives a diagnosis of autism, the doctor may recommend medication or a resource center where the parents can get help for the child. I have yet to see much of anything recommended for the parents. What do you do if the resource center is full and you end up on a waiting list, or there is a fee for the services that you can't afford? What are you supposed to do right now, while you fill out all kinds of paperwork and wait for some assistance?

I recommend Special Intervention Training Techniques (SITT). SITT is the prerequisite foundation for rethinking, reimagining, and reconditioning the misconceptions about autism, while learning how to Be First 2 Respond. Along this journey, I've learned it's difficult to help someone if you haven't developed a sense of mindfulness about who you are and what you are experiencing because of your crisis. It was only possible for me to become better than my best when I realized my very own conditioning and limited thinking. Once I was able to rethink, reimagine, and recondition the way I saw autism, I was able to move forward.

Having a mindfulness presence in the moment allowed me to think about how I was feeling and why. But here is the bonus to using SITT and all the other strategies in this book: you have to become the observer. I recall our college football team watching the footage of a game we'd played the week before. It wasn't so much to see what the other team did; it was to see how we reacted or responded to what was happening in the game. In life, you need to step back and see how are you reacting or responding to your crisis and why. When you become the observer of your life, you have the power to change it.

SITT is so important because when we are faced with a crisis, most of us will focus on the problem and not the solution. During the crisis, we continue to focus on our external environment and search for answers. Instead of focusing on the external factors, we would be better served if we focused on the internal factors. I recommend training attention on the solution. Anytime we look outside ourselves for the answers, we surrender our fate to someone else.

When we search for the answers outside ourselves, we are

depending on someone else to take control over our lives. They literally have control over us. The big question then becomes, who is coming to save you? Here's a hint: no one is coming to save you. The answer is that you are the solution. People don't have time to save you, because they are hoping someone is coming to save them. You have the power within you to create the life you want to live, if only you will take the time to develop yourself.

There are many people with college degrees, rich people, poor people, and people just like you and me who will never take the time to develop and recondition themselves. They didn't teach me this approach in college or on the job. It took my deepest, darkest crisis to beat me down and damn near choke the life out of me for me to realize that, if I ever wanted to see the light of day again and be of any use to my son and to humanity, I had to learn these life strategies for myself the hard way. I am offering you a guide for developing certain skills that will change your life.

SITT is the foundation to every other life strategy in this book. The benefit of comprehending SITT is experiencing a complete change in your life. By understanding these techniques, you will have the possibility of realizing opportunities that you thought were previously closed to you. Once you understand and implement the material discussed in this chapter, you will have the ability to guide your life and your children's lives toward greater success than you previously imagined. SITT offers the building blocks for the vision you have for your future.

The possible consequences for not understanding and implementing SITT include a lack of positive change in your life. Without a SITT foundation, you will continue to make excuses and depend on outside circumstances to free you from yourself.

Only you have the power to free yourself from your preconditioned thoughts and reactions. Without SITT you will have a difficult time envisioning a better future for yourself and your family. When I felt I was dying from my greatest crisis, I couldn't even imagine that light existed. I wasn't thinking clearly during this dark period of my life. I was only following everyone else and getting the same negative results they were getting. I desperately wanted something better for my child.

What does SITT consist of, you ask? Good question. It has five core components, and the first one is mindset. Within the frame of your mind, you have your thoughts, which allow you to think of yourself as the victim or the warrior, as the defeated or the champion. Are you weak or strong, and do you have the tenacity within your mind to overcome your preconditioned negative thoughts? Well, do you?

The second strategy of SITT consists of your effort. How much effort are you willing to exert to improve the quality of your life so that you can improve the quality of your child's life and humanity? You are the only one who can determine how much effort you give to change your circumstances. You don't need a prescription for effort. You need to start with the right mindset.

The third strategy of SITT is adaptability to change, which I believe is where most people suffer the most. Most people do not like change. I am reminded of the saying that everybody wants to go to heaven but nobody wants to die. A lot of people want the miracle but aren't willing to change for it. In order to get the miracle you want, you must be able to adapt to change.

The fourth strategy of SITT is repetition. Every person on the face of the planet has already proven that repetition works. You are where you are in life because of the action that you have consistently repeated over and over again. I suggest that you only repeat what works, which starts with being able to adapt to change.

The fifth and final strategy of SITT consists of not listening to the so-called experts unless they are right. I know we love listening to the so-called experts, but I have found many of them to be shortsighted and completely wrong. The following year there is a new expert and another one the year after that. When we surrender authority to the experts, we tend to become lazy, stop asking questions, and stop searching for what works for us personally.

I believe when a child is diagnosed with autism, the entire family is on the spectrum. We must also think of the well-being of the person raising a child with autism. When Max was diagnosed with autism, there were few resources recommended to us for the benefit of the parents. Everything was for the benefit of our child. I have never been recommended to a training specifically for the person raising a child on the spectrum. As parents, we never received a blueprint of what we should be doing for ourselves in order to help our child.

SITT #1: MINDSET

If you are afraid, then your child will be afraid. It is very easy to become overwhelmed, stressed, and full of anxiety when you first learn your child's diagnosis. Personally, I was thinking that maybe his issue was something else, but not autism. As for the majority of men that I know (including myself), we tend to withdraw and retreat to our man cave. Usually, we are not open about our emotions or forthcoming about how we really feel inside.

As people in general, once we receive bad news, we may want to throw ourselves a pity party. Everyone will react differently to difficult information about their children. We could take that bad news, run with it, and allow it to dictate our lives, or we could allow our greatest crisis to become our greatest miracle. I felt a huge range of emotions and then some. I knew that I had to have the right mindset for our son. I knew that if I showed FEAR and gave in to FEAR, our son would sense it. I didn't want him to grow up being afraid of the world. I had to develop the mindset that exemplified control over my own destiny.

During federal law enforcement training, we were trained to have a certain mindset when conducting an enforcement operation. If we were going to make an arrest, we always took control to make sure our destiny was one that included making it home safely to our families. I remember arriving for an early morning briefing and getting all the details about the person we were going to arrest. After the briefing, we received our assignments and instructions on how this operation would be executed. Most of the time, we had a good understanding of how many people were in the house where the search warrant was being executed. Generally, we knew whether or not the suspect was armed. We had our instructions and were in the right mindset to execute our operation. We had predetermined the time of the execution of the warrant, who would participate, how we would approach the house, and the responsibilities of each person involved. There was always the possibility of unforeseen circumstances. But with the right mindset, we could adapt. When we were prepared with the right mindset, it allowed us to do our job with confidence.

Similarly, people who assisted us with Max knew we were in the right mindset when it came to helping him reach his full potential. If you show your child fear, they will see fear. If you show them everything is going to be all right, then that is what they will see.

When our son was younger, he'd cry when he fell and hurt himself. His mother would pick him up and say, "What's wrong, baby? Did you hurt yourself?" She would comfort him until he stopped crying. Now, when I saw him fall and I knew he wasn't seriously injured, I would tell him, "You're okay. That didn't hurt too badly now, did it?" Usually he would agree and immediately return to playing. We have the greatest influence over our children when they are young and impressionable. They share what we see and feel. I did my best to see the best of our journey, because I wanted Max to see it, too. I did my best to have the right mindset for our day, which turned into our week, which turned into our month, which turned into our years and finally turned out to be our lives.

You can have a mindset of being open to all possibilities by consciously focusing on your daily thoughts. If we are solution-oriented, we usually focus on solutions, which makes us feel in control of our lives and powerful. If we focus on the problem, we feel stress, anxiety, and fear, and usually none of it is productive. Being problem-oriented can drastically disrupt the flow of our mindset.

Fortunately, my mother has a great mindset, and when I was growing up, it was usually positive—until she reached her boiling point with five boys. But overall, she was solution-oriented and I was trained this way my entire childhood. It carried over into my sports, school, career, personal relationships, and professional career. Our children can have the same experience, but we have to give them the opportunity by demonstrating the right mindset for them and for everyone by educating them from a young age.

We practiced having the right mindset for dinnertime education. It is truly a lost art, but I find it to be an invaluable experience. Having a regular dinnertime is a great opportunity for the family to have open discussions about whatever issues they would like to talk about. Most of the time for us, we told funny stories from the past that our son never knew about. We also discussed some serious issues like what was going on in school, what the other children talked about, how Max liked his teachers, whether he had friends, and what he wanted to be when he grew up.

I call this time the best family therapy, because all we do is share what is going on and how we feel while having dinner in the safe environment of our home. It's a great educational opportunity, because we put the cell phones away, all the electronics devices are turned off, and then we go around the table and ask each family member to say three things they are grateful for.

When there was an incident regarding our son, I always asked him what happened, why it happened, and what decision he could make in the future to have a better outcome. I believe in teaching him how to think for himself. I think it is so powerful, considering how little time most parents actually spend talking to their children. We literally spent fifteen years loving, talking, encouraging, motivating, inspiring, influencing, coaching, and training Max to get him where he is today. There was no one method that worked. We tried everything, and we repeated the techniques that worked over and over. Do you recall the last time you and your family had dinner together with no electronic distraction? If not, start today. It is powerful. Many people think that technology is the answer. It has its place, but our children need to learn how to think for themselves and not rely on something or someone else to think for them.

SITT #2: YOUR EFFORT WILL DETERMINE YOUR RESULTS

Once I learned that Max was diagnosed with autism, I knew it would take a lot of effort to help him reach his full potential. I had no idea just how much effort, and I still wasn't sure what the results would be. However, I believed that he deserved the best I could give and then some. I made it my intention to give him the maximum effort that I had.

BE WILLING AND OPEN

First, I had to be willing and open about the effort I was going to put forward. If I gave half-heartedly, then I would receive half-hearted results. I have always come from a belief that if you are going to do something, then you need to put all of your effort into doing it. I have learned there are no shortcuts in life. If you try to take one, you'll get shortcut results. As parents, we don't want shortcut results for our children. When I started, I had no clue as to what I was doing when it came to autism, but I made sure I put forth the effort to learn.

At that time, Max's health was the single most important issue in my life. I made a concerted effort not just to understand autism, but to understand my son as a person. I never wanted to confuse his personality with the typical traits of autism. I always wanted to see him as a person first, even if the rest of the world didn't. That is where I put my effort. I wanted so desperately for the rest of the world to see this beautiful human being who was somewhat socially awkward and learned differently but was also highly intelligent, straightforward, and just as sweet as could be. All I had went into him so that one day, he could reach his best and full potential.

We started out simply playing different games with Max. These were intended to be fun and teach him social, behavioral, and coping skills and, most importantly, self-reliance. I would make a detailed plan as to what I'd do with him during a particular day. I believe that you need a plan, and when you have one, you give it all you got. Once I had detailed what he and I would do for the day, I was totally engaged and fully committed with my effort.

For example, I started coaching him early on in organized basketball. It was a challenging task for both of us, but I believed we'd both benefit from it. Max would have the opportunity to learn something new and to interact with other kids on a regular basis. He would have more exposure and experiences to working as a team with people he just met, which is a useful skill throughout a person's life.

For me, it would be a continuous learning experience that would change the course of my life. If not for this journey, I would not have become the father and human being that I am today. Simply put, the journey with my son made me a better person. I am fortunate to be able to author this book and have the opportunity to share with others that they, too, can allow their greatest crisis to become their greatest miracle. As my effort continued, I could see a difference in our son. Others have often commented on the changes they saw in him over the years. People would ask, "Are you sure he has autism?" and I would reply, "Absolutely."

I understand that most people can't comprehend allowing their greatest crisis to become their greatest miracle, because we have been conditioned to think in a certain way. But I also observed changes in myself. Through my efforts, exposure, and experiences, I became more compassionate. I wanted to do more, not just for my son but also for others who continue to struggle with raising a child with special needs. Caring for someone on the spectrum is not an easy task, but I know I can do more to help people see the beauty and value in all of our children.

MAXIMIZE YOUR EFFORT

Second, I had to learn how to maximize my effort. I believed the best way was to train others who were educating my son on how to give their maximum effort. When we started our son's IEP, I was involved every step of the way. For me, his education wasn't just about being able to repeat information. I wanted him to be able to apply what he had learned and expand on that learning.

I recall when I would take him to the park and have him dribble the basketball. People would comment that he'd be a great basketball player, and I'd say, "Only after he finishes his law degree." To me, it has always been important that our children receive the opportunities they deserve. There should be no preconceived notions that they can't learn and progress. It is up to all of us to reshape the negative narrative about children with autism. I have my quirks about me and I like things a certain way, but that doesn't mean that I can't do the job required of me.

I maximized my efforts by reimagining the story of children with autism in a positive light. If I can bring more humanity to the narrative, then we create a positive ending. The way I decided to approach the IEP was to start with small, reachable goals but not set limits. I viewed the IEP similar to life: we should never limit ourselves regarding what we can accomplish. Now, I had to reshape this narrative for all the experts sitting around the table.

Since I was not an educational expert or a doctor, I had no pre-conceived notions, which meant having no limits for my child. There was some pushback here and there from the school, but once the new narrative started to unfold and the vision was clear, the team was all on board. Then, they started to share more creative ideas about assisting my son with his educational success, which is how I was able to maximize my efforts through resources from the school. I had all of these well-educated experts on my team, and together, we accomplished the miracle that resulted in my son graduating.

INFLUENCE OTHERS

Finally, I had to determine how to influence others so that we all benefited from putting forth maximum effort for a common cause. I thought it would be an easy task, but that wasn't totally accurate. Our son entered school around 2004–2005, and the teachers weren't sufficiently trained about autism in our school district. Sure, there were some special-educational teachers who worked with special-needs kids, but they pretty much lumped everybody together. In order to truly maximize my effort and resources, I had one final strategy: I had to convince my team that the experience they gained from working with Max would benefit other children and their careers personally, while enriching the school and the community.

The teachers working directly with Max were getting firsthand experience about how to teach children on the spectrum. In the beginning, there was resistance, as there usually is when it comes to change, but most people can appreciate the benefits of contributing a great amount of effort. Once I'd reshaped the story for special-needs children for this particular school, I could implement my strategy. We trained the teachers regarding how we worked with our son at home and some of the best educational practices that we stumbled upon as parents.

When you have the right teachers, you have some amazing people who have dedicated their lives to teaching our children life skills that will have an impact on our children forever. They truly deserve a raise and our highest respect. Many times, we ask them to do what we don't do ourselves. And we ask of them to complete this task during the normal class hour while instructing a multitude of other students. Many of the teachers saw the benefits we so vividly described to them. I shared with them there is but one goal, and that is to educate our children so that they are prepared to meet the challenges ahead. Later, teachers would come to appreciate the information and training techniques we'd shared with them as parents.

SITT #3: ADAPTABILITY TO CHANGE

We wanted to give our son the greatest opportunity to be happy, healthy, and successful in life, so I set out to teach him how to be able to adapt to change. Over the years, I have learned firsthand that this adaptability is one of the greatest assets a person can ever acquire. I have met people from around the world, and the happy and successful ones are those able to adapt to change.

Charles Darwin is often paraphrased as saying it is not the strongest or most intelligent of the species that survives but the one that is most adaptable to change.

When Max was diagnosed with autism, I had to adapt to change again. I had to change my perspective about life in order for life to change for me. I am convinced that if a person can adapt to change and view life just a little differently, they will have a greater opportunity to be successful in whatever they do. I had to adapt for my son and for myself. I had to teach him how to adapt to change and to see the world differently. I am amazed by his compassion, intellect, and genuine interest in others.

Today, as a young adult, Max has had more opportunities to adapt to change than I had at his age. I gave him this exposure intentionally. I never tried to solve all of his problems, only to teach him how to think about solutions. If I'd done the work for him, I would have denied him the chance to think for himself and gain new perspective on his challenges. Every day, he is still learning to adapt to change, and so am I. I remember all the hard work that he put into school just so he could keep up academically with the other children. Our children are bright and intelligent, but the schools are not ready to teach them the way they learn best.

Max has excelled in adapting to change. People ask me all the time how we did what we did. In short, we all have our own view of life, and I see value in shifting perspective. We started with the rudimentary skills first, like picking up your toys. We'd tell him if he picked up his toys and put them away, he'd know where they were when he was ready to play with them again. If he liked that idea, he'd comply and put the toys away. If he didn't agree, we'd continue with other reasons to put his belongings away. If we couldn't persuade him, then we used life as the best teacher, because later on, he couldn't find his toys or some were stepped on and broken because he hadn't put them away. We made the most of his days by helping him see the world differently, and we worked on expanding our perspective, too. He was free to participate and observe life and then reach his own conclusion. He has the ability to think for himself and make choices that are conscious and compassionate.

For most of us, change is never easy but always necessary. Now, after his graduation, change is inevitable for the both of us. In fact, a few months before he graduated, I started to notice some shifts in his behavior. He was sleeping a lot (which teenagers do), missing the bus for school, and not all that excited about his upcoming graduation. He just didn't seem focused and interested in school anymore. When I spoke with him about it, he shared with me all his concerns about the new changes about to happen in his life.

He was concerned what would happen to him if he became sick or didn't have money to buy food. I lovingly explained to him that he has a supportive family who will always be there for him. I told him this new chapter in his life is filled with opportunities and possibilities. Ultimately, I decided to take him to speak with an educational psychologist I had met. I spoke with her alone first and shared my concerns. She explained that students who strive for perfection academically have a hard time adapting to change when that particular chapter of their life is over.

She added that those students have become good at what they do and feel very comfortable in their environment. I was somewhat surprised, because this fear is not what I remembered when I graduated from high school. I wanted out of school so badly it wasn't funny. But then again, I wasn't that student reaching for perfection. After meeting with her, Max seemed to be in better spirits, and it just so happens it was time for spring break, so he had a mini vacation. Either way, he was able to tap into his resilience and finish.

To be honest, his graduation represents a big change for me, too. He has been a consistent part of my life for the last eighteen years. Although we strived and dreamed of this day, it still comes with some ambivalence. I am excited for his achievement but also at a loss for words at the end of this chapter of my life. For all of his childhood, I was able to be his guiding shepherd and help him along the way. Now, I must adapt to change, because it's time for him to choose his own path and find his own way.

It's ironic that we hope for days like these for our children but then have a difficult time adapting when they arrive. No matter what we do, we can't stop change, but we can evolve and learn to adapt. God has blessed me with yet another miracle, and I will be glad about it. As a father, I worry about him, but as a life strategist, coach, and trainer, I know he is ready.

SITT #4: REPETITION—FIND OUT WHAT WORKS FOR YOU, AND REPEAT IT AGAIN AND AGAIN

After the initial shock of Max's diagnosis, I asked God what I'd done wrong to have a child with autism. At the time, I didn't know it wasn't a punishment from God but rather a miracle. Through trial and error, I discovered what worked for my son. After I saw the results of some of the strategies I used with him, I reinvested the dividends back into helping him even more. I had to learn early on not to be afraid of failing.

Every time I found a strategy that worked for Max, I repeated it again and again. I made sure he had as much of whatever was working as often as he could. Repetition was the natural response. Once we'd addressed his educational program, I looked at other areas lacking proper training. At the time of his autism diagnosis, he was between two and three years old, which meant I had until he was eighteen or nineteen to figure out how to prepare him for the real world. Many of my strategies would come from my training while playing sports and my years of experience in federal law enforcement.

During football practice, we simulated what it would be like during an actual game. We made some practice days similar to what game day would be like, as realistically as possible. This strategy prepared us for the actual game day and ultimately led us to win the National Championship. I recall all those hot days of practice and then eventually winning the big game. Our repetition prepared us, and our efforts rewarded us.

I took the same approach to improving the quality of Max's life and helping him reach his full potential. As he grew, I made the challenges tougher so he would be prepared for whatever life presented him. Over and over, we would dribble the basketball. Over and over, we would dance to music in the house. Over and over, we would discuss ideas and use our creativity to see life in a different way. Not once has he told me that he was too tired to have fun, which is why I often repeat interesting, exciting, engaging activities over and over with a twist.

When I wanted to increase his vocabulary, I read to him and acted out the events from the book. When I wanted to teach him social skills, I signed him up for team sports. When I wanted to boost his self-esteem, I practiced sports with him. When I wanted to bring out his creativity, I introduced him to art and music. I repeated these strategies over and over for fifteen years. Today, I'm humbled that he trusted me enough to put up with my repetition of getting him prepared for life.

SITT #5: DON'T LISTEN TO THE EXPERTS UNLESS THEY ARE RIGHT

As I mentioned earlier, one of our first doctors told us to give up on our child—but how do you give up on your child? That's not in my DNA. I know that most experts know what they know, but they don't know what they don't know. So I searched for those experts who were looking for answers in places they'd never explored before. In the beginning, I found the same old answers from doctors who were not committed to finding a solution for my child, or any other child for that matter. I was looking for the road of full potential, and most of the doctors just didn't have that vision. I wasn't interested in medicating Max for years on end if it wasn't necessary. I wanted a doctor who was committed to helping Max like their own child, and that, my friend, is a very rare find.

However, I did find one doctor in Phoenix, Arizona, and Max would be the first autistic child he worked with. Dr. Bruce Shelton was the first doctor to give us hope about our son's condition. After Dr. Shelton treated our family and worked with us, he eventually referred us to another brilliant doctor. He said he had taken us as far as he could but knew another specialist who could help us go even farther. I thank Dr. Shelton from the bottom of my heart. Sadly, our family doctor and my friend passed away. He was a great physician, family man, and all-around humanitarian. He gave fully of himself, and I will always be grateful for what he did for our family. If I had listened to the first, pessimistic doctor, I would have never found Dr. Shelton and would not be sharing Max's accomplishments with you.

There is a lot to learn on your journey, so find out as much as you can about your child. You become the expert regarding whatever they're going through. Find the best help for your family that you can learn and grow from. If you find an expert who can't explain how a treatment is going to work and why it should work, keep looking for someone who can. Get to know your child, and do your best in understanding what they are going through when it comes to autism. The situation is not easy for anyone, but it is especially challenging for the child. Let us start with love—you don't need an expert for that.

I recall my high school football years when our coach would tell us to leave it all on the field. He was telling us that to win this simple game (that only a few people came to watch), we needed to be committed and dedicated to winning at all costs. I can still see the fire in my teammates' eyes as we hung on to the coach's every word.

Now, I am telling *you* to leave it all on the field, because tomorrow is not promised and today will surely end. So why are you holding back? Our children are so much more important than a football game, and they deserve everything we have to offer. After many of our games, we would walk off the field looking torn up from the floor up, but when we saw one another, we knew that we had left everything on the field. This is your time and your fight. When it is over, there will be no doubt that we left everything on the field.

You need the mindset of warrior, because we are in the fight for our children's lives, and there is no way we can half-ass this moment. Our effort will show the world we are serious about the health of our children, and our effort is never enough until it is enough. There are always misconceptions and ups and downs in life, so what else is new? Right now, you have the ability to adapt to change. You have consistently proven this over and over.

You want to know how I know? You are reading this book as you continually search for a better way to improve the quality of your child's life. If no one else tells you, then allow me to be the first: you have what it takes. Every morning, repeat it to yourself, because your family is counting on you. When all is said and done, you will be the expert when it comes to your child and you may be the one who goes on to teach and influence others. When you find yourself standing alone, just remember to pray, and I believe your next steps will be guided.

DOS & DON'TS

Do practice SITT.

Do remember you are a warrior fighting for your child's future.

Do leave it all on the field, and I believe you will be a winner.

Don't be afraid to stand alone, because sometimes that's just life.

Don't forget to put forth maximum effort to earn maximum benefit.

Don't forget who you are fighting for—EVER.

CHAPTER ELEVEN

THE POWER OF PRAYER

"Prayer is man's greatest power!"

—W. CLEMENT STONE

MY PRAYER HISTORY

For as long as I can remember, my mother has always prayed, and from the looks of it, her mother prayed all the time, too. I recall my mother saying we have to stay "prayed up." She explained being prayed up meant that you couldn't wait on trouble to happen before praying; you need to pray before trouble begins. I have learned to be prayerful all the time.

Growing up, I spent some nights at my Big Mamma's (my mom's mother) house, and you best believe that if there was an evening church service taking place close by, we were walking over to that service. Prayer has always been a part of my life that was passed on to me from my parents and grandparents. It is my number-one life strategy that I was fortunate enough to be exposed to as a child. I can't say that I always understood the complete meaning of prayer, but I trusted my family members who were teaching it to me. I easily absorbed this strategy as a child, because my mother taught me from a place of love. Her love has followed me into adulthood, and I learned the meaning of prayer during my life journey.

I recall the summers that I stayed at my Big Mamma's house. Each night, we would say the Lord's Prayer together at bedtime, which is how I first started to pray. It didn't make much sense to me then, but because I respected my Big Mamma, I knew not to talk back and I prayed with her. I was old enough to know that what she was teaching me was what she believed, and it more than likely had sustained her through some difficult times. Little did I know at that time that this simple yet powerful prayer would have a significant impact on my life.

Our parents taught us to pray and always to be prayerful. We prayed before every meal, we prayed before bedtime, we prayed when our parents got a raise at work, and my mom prayed all through my high school years, repeatedly asking God to help me listen in school so that I would graduate. God is good, because I graduated with my high school senior class and then went on to college.

In this chapter, I want to share with you my personal life experiences with prayer, which includes how I pray, the art of being thankful, the best time to pray, why you should pray, and what you should pray for. If you are willing and open to exploring with me for a few paragraphs, I will explain to you why I still pray every day.

For me, prayer is a way of life that increases my growth in faith and guides me to live a more balanced life. The power of prayer has strengthened me at all levels, and I believe the power of prayer can strengthen you as well. Simply put, the benefits of prayer are miraculous. When you are prayerful, the entire universe is available to help you reach your destiny.

The consequences of not being prayerful may result in you setting limitations on what you believe you can accomplish in your life. See, when you are prayerful, you don't have to be wishful. The power of prayer can help you build resilience, and with resilience, you have the ability to bounce back from a crisis. The power of prayer doesn't mean that your desires are going to come the way you think they should come, but they're coming. The pitfalls of not being prayerful are that you diminish your hopes and desires as they relate to the life God has planned for you. I don't know if a person can truly believe in miracles without being prayerful. I believe the two go hand in hand. I also believe it's common to think small and live small if we are not prayerful. The power of prayer allows you to believe that miracles are possible.

Nike is known for its famous logo and the slogan "Just Do It." When I was a child, I just did it, because it's what my parents taught me to do. Just pray. It doesn't matter where you are in your life at this moment, because God loves you and will never leave you. Prayer is always available to us, and I believe it is one of the greatest powers that we have. Over the years, my faith has been shaken many times, but through prayer, my faith was strengthened. During the tough times, I was able to hold on just a little while longer, and God blessed me with what I needed, when I needed it, to continue on my journey. God can do the same for you when you use the power of prayer.

HOW DO I PRAY?

I am always encouraged by this passage from the Bible in Matthew 7:7–8: "Ask, and it shall be given you; seek, and ye shall find; knock, and it shall be opened unto you: For every one that asketh receiveth; and he that seeketh findeth; and to him that knocketh it shall be opened."

For most of my adult life, I have used several forms of prayer. To be honest, I am probably just like most people in asking God for a lot of things all the time. During my darkest period with our son's autism diagnosis, I was always asking God for help, good doctors, good schools, and a good night's rest. You get the picture. I was asking for everything.

Remember that God knows your need before you request it, but it is also powerful to humble yourself before God and ask for what you need. I believe that God is waiting to bless us according the scripture above when it says, "Ask, and it shall be given you." Have you tried prayer today? When was the last time that you asked God to help you? It doesn't matter where you are in life, nor does it matter the last time you spoke to God. He is waiting to hear from you today. God is ready to bless you, so start asking in order to receive.

The next form of prayer that I use is mindfulness mediation, during which I prepare my mind, body, and spirit to listen to God. I have found it extremely helpful to listen to what God is telling us. The above scripture further reads, "Seek, and ye shall find." When I prepare myself for mindfulness mediation, I take a moment to find a quiet place, slow down my breathing, clear my mind, and open my heart so I can seek what God is telling me. I am totally focused in the present moment, and my thoughts and emotions are all with God. At this point, I am not asking for anything, because I am actively listening to God speak to me.

This form of prayer can be done throughout the day or as needed. I have noticed that when I practice mindfulness mediation before starting my workday, the day goes so much better and I experience less stress. I have also noticed that when I practice mindfulness meditation before going to bed, I sleep better and wake up totally refreshed. When I meditate on what God is telling me, I am certain that I am headed in the right direction.

THE ART OF BEING THANKFUL

Being thankful to God for the blessings that He has already given me while He continues to bless me is a powerful affirmation of prayer. This thankfulness can become very emotional and intense. Affirming prayer is one of my favorites, and here's why. When I go to God in prayer, I am coming from a thankful heart. It is that feeling of gratitude that fills me with joy. When my heart is filled with joy, I literally do not have the capacity to be worried or concerned about anything else. This affirmation of prayer reduces my stress and guides my mind to a positive perspective on life. When I am thankful to God for all the blessings I've received, I see life completely differently and live it differently. When you are thankful to God, you should live as though you are thankful. I believe being thankful to God allows your inner world to be reflected in your outer world. Personally, life is just more beautiful when I am thankful.

For me, having a sense of thankfulness for what God has already blessed me with is more than enough to be happy about, yet I know God is continuing to bless me more and more each and every day. Being thankful means having faith that God has heard the knock and will answer your prayers. The passage above reads, "Knock, and it shall be opened unto you." You can start knocking today by being thankful to God.

I have discovered that when I am thankful and counting my blessings, I don't have time to focus on negativity. Finding something in your life to be thankful for increases your opportunity to realize the many blessings you already have. It is a powerful mindset to be thankful and to show gratitude to God, which translates into living a life of prosperity.

Every day of my life, I do my best to thank God for the blessings He has already bestowed upon me. I thank God long before I visually see any results of a miracle in my life, because I have faith that He has already set in motion that which is necessary to grant me my miracle. As I reflect on my life, I am reminded there is not one time that God has left me stranded. I have not lived a perfect life, but still God has always been there for me, and He is here for you.

I encourage you to write in your journal all that you are thankful for and see if it doesn't outweigh your troubles. For the troubles you are going through, ask God for a miracle and then thank God that He has already blessed you with whatever you prayed for.

THE BEST TIME TO PRAY

Here is the short answer regarding the best time to pray. The best time for prayer was yesterday, a better time for prayer is today, and a still great time for prayer is tomorrow. Simply put, all the time is the best time for prayer. When the doctor advised us to give up on Max, I remember his mother tearfully asking me if I thought Max would be okay. With all the faith I could muster in my heart, I said I believed he would.

The best time for prayer was yesterday because all of us will experience a crisis at some point during our lives. If you haven't experienced a crisis yet, just keep on living. It is not necessary to wait and experience a crisis before you begin to pray. In fact, I recommend that you start practicing prayer in your life right now. It doesn't matter what you are going through; prayer is one of the most powerful ways to sustain and change your life.

Upon learning Max had autism, I immediately turned to prayer, because I knew its power. I had a reference point because I come from a praying family. When I began to pray for Max and our entire family, my situation didn't suddenly improve overnight. In fact, it was quite the opposite. It seemed like things just got worse. At times, it seemed like life wouldn't get any better. I believe if you really want your life to improve, you must put forth effort to make it happen. The same is true of prayer. You have to put in effort. I believe you have to open your heart and mind and allow the power of prayer to guide you.

Sometimes, we think circumstances will happen one way, and when they don't go the way we think they should, we wonder why God didn't answer our prayers. If we don't open our hearts and minds, we will always think God didn't answer our prayers. When you pray, you must believe and be open and willing to receive God's blessings.

A better time for prayer is today, because change doesn't come easily. Prayers may not be answered right away. It will take some practice for you to open your heart and mind to be prepared for your blessings. I encourage you to pray today and continue to put forth the effort each and every day through your prayers. I believe if you continually put effort into your prayers, change will come. Many people prayed for Max, and it was a very slow process to see change happening. I implore you not to give up; not seeing the change right away doesn't mean it's not in the process of happening. In fact, you may not be the first person to see the benefits of your efforts, because you are too close to the situation. Just keep praying today, and change is going to come.

I've shared with you many examples about Max in this book. I found myself praying all the time, and when I met other parents of children diagnosed with autism, I'd ask them if they'd tried prayer. I like to share with others what I believe to be one of our greatest powers.

In fact, the Bible teaches us in Proverbs 3:5–6, "Trust in the Lord with all your heart, and lean not on your own understanding; in all your ways acknowledge Him, and He shall direct your paths." When we started this journey as a family, we had no understanding about autism, but we trusted in the Lord and received our miracle.

Finally, I believe a great time for prayer is tomorrow, because maybe I forgot to ask God for all that I needed the day before. I believe we should be persistent with our prayers, not because we believe God didn't hear our prayers or forgot about us but to increase our faith and to prepare our hearts and minds to receive the goodness of God. I also think that when you find yourself having doubts—and we all have doubts—you must remain prayerful with the understanding that tomorrow is a new day. With a new day comes new opportunities. After a while, the continuation of prayer slowly began to affect how I saw life. The darkness was no longer dark, and the sweet rays of sunshine were peeking through the shadows that surrounded me. Pray now and remain prayerful while patiently waiting for change in our lives.

WHY PRAY?

I believe sincere prayer comes from love. Other people often ask me what is the best treatment we have provided for Max, and without an ounce of doubt, I tell them it has been love. From love, I could see the transformation in his behavior as he slowly came out of his shell to join the rest of the world. I also noticed my own transformation and the way I started to approach my crisis.

As I continued to pray, my faith strengthened with the belief that God was in the process of blessing my family with a miracle. Prayer added fuel to my determination to improve the quality of life for Max. I prayed because I needed the fuel that prayer provided me in order to get through another day. Many days, prayer energized me emotionally, and it was like a cleansing of my entire body knowing that I had given my burden over to God.

I believe prayer is one of the most powerful acts that we can learn to do. I was very fortunate, because my Big Mamma taught me the Lord's Prayer, my mother preached the power of prayer, and God showed me the miracle of prayer. I know I have greatly benefited from my mother's prayers and the prayers of many others.

As I reflect on my life's blessings, I can truly appreciate what has been bestowed upon me. I am grateful for the power of prayer and am humbled by all who took the time to pray for my family and me. I will never know all of the people by name who took a moment of their precious life to be a blessing to me. I am thankful that these individuals thought enough of me to say a prayer for me.

There is always a reason to pray, but during our journey from Autism 2 Awesome, I prayed to be guided on how to help improve Max's life. In the end, he became a highly accomplished and well-traveled student, in addition to being an all-around wonderful human being who brought light to my life and the lives of many people at his school and in our community.

Personally, I am prayerful because it's a way of life for me. I can't imagine my life without prayer. I was exposed to this practice at a very early age, and it has proven to be the best strategy I know to tap into the greatness within. Prayer is my moment to express my thoughts, desires, fears, doubts, and concerns to God and God alone, allowing me to focus on what's important in my life. It also gives me an opportunity to be a blessing to someone else by praying for them.

I pray because it strengthens my day-to-day resolve to move forward in a positive way. Learning that Max had autism was overwhelming, and we were determined to find a solution to improve the quality of his life and help him reach his full potential. Because of the struggles and difficulties of raising a child with autism, it is easy to give up. I know because I have been there, and at some point in time, a lot of people have experienced the feeling of wanting to give up.

Prayer can get you through that moment of disappointment and build your resolve and determination to help you keep on keeping on. There have been so many times that I have felt down and out, but like the song goes, I'm gonna have a little talk with Jesus and tell him all about my problems. I feel better just knowing I have someone to tell my problems to and having the belief that I'll get over this struggle. Think about how much better you feel when you can share your problems with a friend and they say, "I'll be praying for you." Prayer is powerful. When you tell your problems to God, help is already on the way.

For me, the power of prayer is a huge stress reliever that allows my thoughts to be more solution-oriented. Prayer allows me to be consistent, too, and here is I what I mean. When you sincerely go to God in prayer, it's best to go with the belief that your prayer will be answered. Otherwise, why pray? When I pray, I have the belief that God has already answered my prayer, which helps me become consistent in my thoughts, beliefs, and actions. Are you living better than your best, with the belief your prayers have already been answered? I encourage you to tap into your greatness within through prayer and to live as though your prayers have already come true.

WHAT SHOULD YOU PRAY FOR?

What you choose to pray for is totally up to you, but I will share with you what I prayed for when I was experiencing my deepest, darkest life crisis.

I prayed for a miracle…and here is why. Max was diagnosed with autism, and we didn't know anything about autism. We were overwhelmed for many reasons, and our emotions were scattered all over the place. As parents, we were in a vulnerable state of mind and desperate for a solution. During this dark period of our life, we knew we needed a miracle from God. So I prayed for one. I had no idea what the miracle would look like, but I desperately needed God's intervention. I didn't know when the miracle would happen, but I believed that God heard my prayers and would bless me with a miracle.

As I continued to pray, I was guided to be more specific as to what I wanted from God. I started asking God just to help me help Max. I really believe that we learn the most when we are faced with the most difficult challenges of our lives. When it is make-or-break-us time, the human spirit is incredible. I'd suddenly have epiphanies about what to do next for Max, and I knew it was God answering my prayers. Prayer allowed me to be open to all possibilities, which in turn provided many more solutions.

In the beginning, I was just trying to hang on to my sanity. Then, I began to ask God for strength in what was by far the toughest battle of my life. I knew I would not achieve an overnight victory, because within this crisis, there were many lessons for me to learn. I have always enjoyed helping others, but at that time, I would become impatient. I have learned to be more compassionate to all people, because we are all on a journey of learning. I have come to appreciate the human spirit of all people, because each one of us has our own personal story and inner strength waiting to be tapped into. You may not yet realize that you have it, but you do. You just need to learn how to tap into it, and prayer can help get you there.

As I reflect back over my life, there is not one time that God has left me, and He will never leave you, either.

As I continued on my journey, God blessed me with knowledge and then with wisdom regarding how to share my new knowledge. I was introduced to books that I didn't know existed, and we started to discovered doctors who were literally a Godsend.

Many people understand that physical exercise is good for you. Prayer was my spiritual exercise and propelled me from one day to the next. Prayer was my go-to, to get up, get going, and keep going. I discovered the miracle we so desperately seek is rooted in prayer. Unlike any other species on this planet, we can express our thoughts, desires, and frustration to our creator, who is waiting to bless us. All we have to do is take the first step. So I made prayer an integral part of every day to improve the quality of our family's life. I made it a way of life, and I have been blessed beyond measure.

I always remember to say a prayer for others. We are all connected in some shape, form, or fashion. Many people are going through a crisis right now, and you have just learned about the power of prayer. You have the power to bless someone else right now, and in doing so, I believe that you will be blessed. When you find yourself deep in prayer, remember there is more than enough to go around for the entire world. Your prayers can make a difference in the world today, and we need all the prayers we can get.

When we begin to live our lives according to the scripture from Matthew, then there is nothing that is impossible through the power of prayer. I encourage you to use the power of prayer in your life. It is always a good time to pray, and what you choose to ask for is totally up to you. If you don't know what to pray for, simply ask God to show you the way. Always give thanks, because we all have been blessed simply by being here. I believe when we choose to use the power of prayer, we can transform our lives, and our hopes for tomorrow can become our reality today.

DOS & DON'TS

Do pray for a miracle if that is what you want.

Do stay prayed up, because prayer is so powerful.

Do be thankful, because there is so much to be thankful for.

Don't forget to pray for others, because none of us can do all of it alone.

Don't be discouraged if your prayers are not answered right away.

Don't forget to ask for what you want.

CHAPTER TWELVE

ONE DAY

"One day spent with someone you love can change everything."

—MITCH ALBOM

The day we were told about Max's autism sent our lives into a total tailspin. It would take a moment or two for us as parents to process the reality of what autism is and the ramifications it would have on our lives. At first, we were hopeful as we began our research, but then we were devastated all over again. Life would continue with the ups and downs while we dreamt of our situation one day improving.

Life gets better when we make it get better. Some say life "is what it is," but I believe it is what we make of it. This chapter covers why it's important to understand that all we have is one day, and that one day is today. What we do with it makes all the difference in the world. We have one day to love and one day to cry, one day to live and one day to die. Choose this one day to live, and choose to love.

Not fully understanding this concept means missing opportunities to experience love. I love Max so much that I didn't see autism—I saw *him*. I see a child who needs love and understanding, which we all could use more of, including me. I encourage you not to miss the beauty of living life in the moment. For me, there is nothing more important in life than experiencing love. I am so fortunate that God placed Max in our lives so that I could experience and appreciate the love of our son.

In this chapter, I will share with you the hopes and dreams that we longed for during our most difficult days. In addition, I will tell you how self-reflection was instrumental for me to realize that my one day was today. Now, because of what our journey together has taught me, I am able to teach others. And here is what is so incredible about my teaching journey: the more I teach others, the more I learn from others. I believe it's important for each one to teach one.

I encourage you to keep going. There will be many difficult challenges, but keep going anyway. Your one day is closer than you think, but you have to believe it. Finally, I will share with you that Max is all grown up and doing extremely well, but we never stop being parents. The strategies I developed along the way are here for you to use as a guide to reach your one day.

THE DREAM

Like many other people who have children diagnosed with autism, I often thought about what life would be like one day for Max. I wondered if he'd one day reach his fulfillment, if he'd get married one day and have his own children, if he'd one day speak in full sentences, and whether the temper tantrums would stop. (I thought about this last one a lot.)

There is no known definitive cause of autism, but there are

plenty of misconceptions about it. However, we have this one day to start reshaping and reimagining our story into a new reality and managing the conditions of autism. We do so one day at a time. I found myself living in the future and too many "one days" were passing me by. I couldn't afford to live in the future, and our son couldn't afford to wait for me to return to the present. I had to allow my one day to become my today. I was going to do everything in my power one day at a time to make the very most out of my life to benefit Max's life.

Many days, I was living in the future and missing out on the present moment. I was missing out on the gift that had been given to me. Max was perfect just as he was, which made each and every one of my days an absolute miracle. For the longest time, I was convinced that I was teaching him. Then it dawned on me that Max was teaching me. I thought he had special needs, but I didn't think that I also had special needs. Our son blessed me with the opening of my heart to love and joy. There he was, my gift. Doctors couldn't explain it, and most people didn't want to talk about it, but the love and compassion that our children have can change our world.

Dreams are important, and I encourage you to have big dreams. But remember to live each and every day in the moment. When we live in the moment, the future is not some distant place that we hope to reach one day. We have the opportunity to experience and appreciate the journey of reaching our dreams. When we live in the moment, we are living our dreams, and everything after that moment is simply an extension of them.

If we are always dreaming, then we may never get to where we would like to be, because we can't remember where we started. Instead, we can dream and see every day is the process of our dreams becoming our reality, because today is part of the dream. I didn't wake up one morning and find everything that I wanted was accomplished. I woke up each day appreciating life and feeling thankful for the opportunity to have this one day to live in my dream and not out of it.

Most people live their lives outside of their dreams. They dream of becoming this or that but never do anything about it. You have the power within you to live your dream today. One day, our son only spoke two words, so I read to him and we listened to music to help increase his vocabulary. Today, he speaks two languages and uses words that I don't understand. It was my dream that he would one day speak more than two words, but each day before this dream became a reality, I loved the moments we read together. I cherish the moments we played "tickle time" together, and I can't tell you how many times I massaged his feet so he would fall asleep. Those times are distant memories now, but they all played a very important role in living our dreams.

REFLECTION

One day as I reflected on our lives, I started to allow my one day to become my today. I coached Max many times when he played basketball, which helped him learn some life skills. It also taught me a few as well. I believe there is something that we can learn from each individual. My journey with Max taught me love and patience and made me a better human being.

Those days of practicing basketball together allowed us to build a bond that continues until this day. The strategies he learned when he didn't want to go to basketball practice taught him discipline, which led to him understanding that you have to continue to do your best in order to get what you want out of life. Those one days add up to a surprising life of miracles, starting with the small steps of talking about practice and how to respect your teammates and opponents while still putting forth all your effort to win the basketball game. We learned when you put forth your best effort, you actually help make the other person better. I remember at those first practices, Max was like a fish out of water.

Almost every kid on the court was better than he was athletically. Actually, they all were better than he was in basketball. During those days, I would explain to him that we all have gifts, and in those areas where we may not be as gifted as others, we have to work a lot harder. I knew one day, he would grow up and leave home. When that one day came, I wanted him to be prepared. I knew I only had so many days before I would no longer be his basketball coach and able to give him instructions. That one day has arrived sooner than I anticipated. I knew it was coming; I just didn't know it would come so fast. I really miss those days. When I was living those days, they were tough and time-consuming. Today, though, I see the results of all the hard work and am glad we had those moments in time to share all of the experiences that made us who we are.

Having graduated from high school, he will start to make more and more of his own decisions. One day, he will have his first job, girlfriend (OMG), wife, and family. For me, one day will seem like a lifetime ago and yet only yesterday. There is only one way I know to overcome the one-day illusion, which is to live today. I knew one day he would be an adult out in the world and I wouldn't be there for him. So I began teaching others what I had learned along the way. If your path crosses with my son's, please show him love, because he learned to show it to others. I promise that if we cross paths, I will show you and your family love, too. Imagine what the world would be like if each of us would take one day to show love to one another.

EACH ONE TEACH ONE

First, I started to teach other parents and also developed a special program for fathers. I knew there was no way I could do this work alone, so I had to make the most of my limited opportunities. While I was working as a U.S. diplomat in Lagos, Nigeria, I attended the Annual Autism Conference there. The conference was in its infancy then but has since grown into something meaningful and impactful. It provides hope and sound advice for families. I was impressed by the very first one I attended. I continued to be consistent and got involved to see what I could offer. I must say the Nigerians were well on their way to allowing their one day to become their today.

I personally witnessed them being the change they wanted to see in the world. The conference had some powerful local Nigerian speakers, and the information was insightful. I was happy to attend because I saw that resources in Nigeria could be hard to come by when compared to some other countries. The Nigerians made it work, and attending was an awesome experience for me. I started speaking at a few events in Nigeria, which gave me a different perspective regarding the way I was approaching my training. Every person's needs and available resources are different, so I had to relate to each person in different countries in a way that was realistic.

Our Autism 2 Awesome training in Nigeria was well received. The Nigerians built a community of individuals who came together collectively and generated more awareness and training around autism. The autism community in Nigeria started to teach one another what they had learned, and the knowledge started to spread with amazing results.

I am often asked where to start, and I say just start. Once you start, you'll see what changes you need to make in order to make your efforts better. When it came to Max, as his parents, we simply got started to improve the quality of his life. By doing so, he improved the quality of our lives. When I first started chasing him around the house with that big exercise ball, I had no idea what it would lead to, but I knew he enjoyed me chasing him with it. When I started, I didn't know what skills I would be teaching him or what I would learn from it. The most important step is to start teaching our children what we know and allow them to teach us what they need. Remember, like Nike...just do it.

When Max participated in a recreational basketball league, it raised more awareness in the community where you wouldn't normally see kids on the spectrum playing sports. People noticed that Max was different when he was playing, and they would be nice and cordial about his limited skills. What they didn't realize at the time is that I was teaching him life skills. Basketball is a game to go play and have fun. You don't have to take it too seriously. Sometimes, other people are going to be better than you in certain areas; take the opportunity to learn from them. The simple act of getting our son involved in a recreational basketball league made the community more aware and open regarding their own children with special needs. Everyone has the opportunity to learn and to become more inclusive when they are exposed to different experiences.

One day, I had a conversation with the parent of a child I was coaching. I'd noticed that her son had similar characteristics to Max's. I asked her how her son liked playing basketball, and she said he loved it. Then she added, "You know, he has been diagnosed with autism." I said I didn't know. I was glad to see that she got started with enrolling him in activities with other children. Later, I started to notice more and more children with similar autism traits on my basketball team. I never asked the parents if they were on the spectrum, because I was there to teach them life skills while having some fun playing basketball. The community was becoming more and more aware of children on the autism spectrum, and they all played together and had fun.

KEEP GOING

I am amazed by how much Max has learned over the years, because I wondered every day if he understood what I was trying to teach him. He probably wondered the same about me. If I was going to allow my one day to become today, I had to keep going and be consistent. If I was going to listen to Gandhi and be the change I wanted to see in the world, then I had to educate others and myself on a regular basis about reshaping the lives of our children with autism. There was so much to be done, and I got excited knowing I had this small power to help change the lives of others.

I developed a consistent routine with coaching Max how to play the game of basketball. Then one day when the season ended, parents rushed to me and asked, "Coach Kerry, are you coaching the next session of basketball?" I said, "Yes, why?" They said they wanted their children to play for me again. I thought to myself, *Wow*. I had no idea. I told them there are good coaches for the other teams as well. The parents said, "My child likes to play for you, because you made it fun and they learned a lot."

That's when I developed my other program, Ballin' 4 Autism, to teach kids life strategies through sports.

If Max didn't want to go to practice, I reminded him that once he was older and got a job, if he didn't go to work, he wouldn't get paid. Then I added that if you don't get paid, then you don't have food to eat and can't pay for a place to live. I would tell him, "We all have bad days, but today is not one of them. Now get your shoes on, because we are late for practice." I taught him that if he wanted to get better at anything, he had to keep going and be consistent. I added that you can't practice basketball only once a week and expect to be your best. You must continue to train in order to get better at it. I learned these principles from living my life and accomplishing my goals.

ALL GROWN UP

Today, Max is a young man and standing on solid ground. He is capable of doing a lot, but most importantly, he can think for himself. He has the opportunity to reach his fulfillment if he continues to learn and take one day at a time.

I want to help others reach their fulfillment as well. To make my one day my today, I personally focused on what was most important to me at that time. During Max's childhood, the most important issue was his health. I was motivated because I knew if I lived in the moment, change would come over time. Now, my one day has become my today.

Living in the moment and embracing each experience guided me to help Max reach his fulfillment. I am so proud of him for believing in me, even though I didn't know what I was doing at first, to help prepare him for the world. Each day taught me something different and prepared me for the next day. Every moment was a teaching and training opportunity for both of us. I tried to make it fun, but that can't always be done. I had to do what I had to do.

In addition, to make sure I stayed in the moment, I used some of the other tools I described earlier in the book. I used my journal to tell myself exactly what I was going to do and when. I made myself a schedule, because success was that important to me. Research has shown that people who write their goals down are more likely to accomplish them than people who don't write their goals down. Writing strategies down made it easier for me to keep up with life and remain committed to Max's health.

One day, I wanted to educate law enforcement personnel on how to respond and de-escalate situations involving individuals on the spectrum. In 2011, just before I was reassigned to Lagos, Nigeria, as a United States diplomat I trained over 200 law enforcement personnel regarding autism. The training was well received. I remember one officer approaching me afterward and saying, "When I heard that you would be speaking about autism, I thought to myself, 'What do I need this for?'" However, having finished the training, he said, "I am going to talk to my chief about having you come to our department to train all of our officers. I never knew all of this stuff you were telling us." I thanked him and got similar remarks from other participants in the class.

A little while later, I received a telephone call from the Phoenix Police Department in Arizona. They informed me that they were producing a video on mental illness and wanted to know if I would participate in it and talk about autism. I did, and the video was released to over 15,000 first responders in Arizona. I love sharing this knowledge and helping others so we can create a community that makes life better for all of us. After being in Nigeria and getting involved, I was asked to conduct my training for fathers, which was also well received. I have been blessed in so many ways, and it is yet another blessing for me to share with others.

Remember to make your one day a reality today. Always have your dreams, but live in your dreams each moment and not outside of them. Reflecting on your life is a good way to live in the moment. Take time to teach others what you have learned and inspire them to keep going. One day, our children will be all grown up, so live and love today. Life has taught me never to give up. One day, I thought about writing a book about my journey with Max, and wouldn't you know it? I have written a book. My one day is today, because our family never gave up. My prayer is that you will never give up, either.

DOS & DON'TS

Do have big dreams—the bigger, the better.

Do teach others so we all can benefit.

Do love and live in the moment.

Don't live outside of your dreams, because you have the power to make them a reality.

Don't live in the future, because life is to be lived now.

Don't stop.

CHAPTER THIRTEEN

NEVER GIVE UP

"No child is un-teachable. I will never give up on any kid. Every child can learn."

—SUSANA MARTINEZ

To put it mildly, I was a bad little kid. I mean *bad*. Looking back, I drove my mother crazy, but she never gave up on me. She always told me that I could do great things if I would put my mind to it and just do my best. By far, I received more disciplinary actions from my parents than all my other siblings combined. Through all of my struggles in school, along with my uncooperative (delinquent) behavior as a teenager, my mother never gave up on me…ever. As I reflect on the years gone by, I will always be grateful that she stood by me.

There are many benefits to not giving up, so read and reread this chapter as many times as necessary. When you never give up, there are opportunities waiting for you just ahead. They're called blessings, and they come from the goodness of God. The benefits of never giving up strengthen us every day. Our daily struggle can build us up or tear us down, but if you never give up and never give in, you'll only grow stronger. Never giving up serves as a great example to our children that instills in them the importance of showing up every day, ready to put the work in.

As usual with life, there is a flip side. There are dire consequences for giving up. Our football coach used to tell us if we quit, then we'd always be a quitter. Personally, I believe once you give up the first time, it is easy for you to give up the next time. Sure, there have been plenty of times that I wanted to give up, but the love that I have for Max would not allow me to. One of the dire consequences of giving up is that you may never know your true potential or that of your child. Another dire consequence is that you may live a life of regret and see yourself as a failure. I have never met a person who quit on something important to them and did not have some regret.

In the following pages, I will admit persistence is hard. This is not a secret. If it were easy, there would be no need for me to write this book or for you to read it. It's important to get everyone involved in the journey, which is why I explain in these pages what daddies can do. All of us have got to pitch in, because this struggle is too important. In order to help our children fulfill their potential, we must be firm but flexible. Lastly, I will share with you how to never give up.

IT'S HARD

During our crisis, there were many hard days to get through, and it seemed like the struggle would never end. Many times, I just tried to hang on until the next day. I knew the crisis would end one day and I would be stronger because it. I now look at Max and see how wonderful he is doing in life, and I thank God for giving me the strength to never give up. Then I think to myself, what if I had given up on him like the doctor told me to? I think about the times when we tried different life strategies for him and nothing seemed to be working. We as parents had to muster up enough motivation to try another tactic, still uncertain if it would work. Did I mention that it's hard?

Compared to when Max was first diagnosed with autism not so long ago, times have changed somewhat with regard to getting information. There are many more resources available, and we have read about children with autism leading fulfilling and productive lives. I think there is more hope available today than in years past, and we all can use a little bit more hope. If I had taken the doctor's advice and given up on Max, I would not be writing this book today. Because of the journey that we shared as a family, I have learned so much about how to help him, how to help others, and also how to help myself. I never knew writing my story would be so therapeutic for me. There was so much pain that I didn't have time to feel during our crisis, and writing this book dredged up some powerful emotions.

Personally, this book represents a healing step and a new chapter in my life. I know I have done the best I could for Max. I made plenty of mistakes and lost some opportunities, but we must never give up. Today may not be perfect, but tomorrow might be just a little bit better. If we give up, we will never know. I always had to remember it wasn't just my life that would be impacted if I gave up. I was impacting the life of our son, who was not in a position to help himself. I would also affect others who need this book to overcome their first-step fears. I owed him a better life, and he didn't care what my background was, my economic status, the color of my skin, and certainly not my educational level. He wanted and needed his father's love.

WHAT CAN DADDIES DO?

When daddies are involved in their children's lives, they can have a huge impact on the child's success now and later. As a daddy, I wanted to show Max every day that I loved him unconditionally. I wanted to show him that he was already special and didn't have to do anything additional to earn my love. Giving up never really entered my mind, only how to keep going. I would remind myself to keep going when I would look at him and see how beautiful of a being he was. Forget about what they call "autism," because I saw him as a gift from heaven, and our journey together would be a blessing for us both.

Daddies can put the work in every day and teach our children what we know. I believe we all have gifts, and daddies can share those gifts with the autism community. We can toss the ball, read a book, sing a song, teach carpentry, give foot massages, cook a meal, attend parent-teacher conferences, or start a father support group. All of these actions add up to our children having better life experiences. Daddies can support their spouses, because this journey is an emotional roller coaster that's easier to handle when we have someone to share our screams (I'm sorry, I meant *dreams*) with.

I know if I had given up on Max, I would be living my latter days on earth with a lot of regret. I would have never known his true potential, because I never put the work in. As a dad, I knew I had to help improve the quality of Max's life. Had I not done so, I would have never known my true potential, either. Never giving up meant I couldn't be a spectator in life. I had to get involved. You have to do what will make a difference in someone else's life. Never choose a doctor, a friend, or an acquaintance who encourages you to give up. Nobody knows what the future holds for you and your family, and they certainly don't know what it holds for you if you persist through the difficult times.

At first it was slow going when I signed Max up for soccer, but my motto is if we start something, we are going to finish it. He didn't like the afternoon heat during practice, but he was okay with the cooler Saturday morning games. He also enjoyed the snacks and the juice boxes that the parents purchased for the team to share. We stuck with it, and then I started to see him become more involved with his teammates, which was one of my reasons for getting him started in sports.

We were able to cultivate his social and behavior skills through sports. From playing sports, Max had the opportunity to expand his communication skills by using language with children his own age. I noticed he followed instructions better, and this skill transferred into the classroom. Without all these activities we shared together, I never would have had the opportunity to learn and create these life strategies to pass on to other families.

BE FIRM BUT FLEXIBLE

At times, I witnessed Max mimicking the behavior of others. When it was positive behavior, we encouraged and reinforced it. When he started mimicking negative behavior, we explained to him why it was inappropriate and redirected him to more positive options. We never gave up on correcting his behavior, because we knew that over time, he would understand. The different sports practices and games were little life lessons along the way that we all could learn from. Sports are the greatest activities that I know to learn the attitude of never giving up. We had to be firm but flexible when we were teaching him right from wrong. We discussed with him the way other people might feel and why it is not nice to intentionally make other people feel bad.

Most children love to play and be involved with games, make

friends, laugh, and have fun. I think we learn best when we are having fun, and everyone can be involved. Having fun is a natural state for kids to learn to make small decisions, including about what games they would like to play, who is going be on the same team, and what the rules are.

Participating in sports prepares us for the future. The journey taught me that I have the know-how to help others, because Max has taught me so much along the way. I never would have had the opportunity if I had given up. During this journey, I learned just as much about myself as I did about autism. If I had given up, I would have missed out on learning and doing more. It feels great to accomplish your goals, but there is no better satisfaction than helping others accomplish theirs.

In addition, I would encourage Max never to give up during each practice session and to work a little harder to get better at any sports activity. I was striving for him to develop his mental capacity and challenge himself and never to give up just because he wasn't the best at something. I wanted him to cultivate the never-give-up attitude for sports, school, career, and life. Many parents of children with special needs want to protect them from any difficulties. I wanted Max to learn to persist through the difficult times and take care of himself and his family when the time came.

He has faced many challenges without ever giving up. He can take care of himself. He has completed advanced courses, learned a second language, experienced different cultures, and traveled the world. He is well on his way to making a positive impact on others. I wouldn't have missed this journey with him for the world, and if I had listened to that doctor, I would have lost the opportunity to see my little boy become a capable young man.

HERE'S HOW TO NEVER GIVE UP

In my darkest moments, I lived in fear of the unknown and was uncertain about what to do next. Then, I discovered one life strategy, which led me to another. For the first time in a long time, I felt something come alive inside of me. I began to gain courage and strength as my life perspective started to change. It was finally a new day for me as I began using these new life strategies each and every day. They guided me toward multiple ways to improve the quality of Max's life and improved my life as well.

I humbly share the strategies with you in this book. There are many ways for you to embrace and learn how to never give up. If you work the strategies, the strategies will work for you. I suggest that you start with one that you feel you can try right away, and embrace a second strategy when you are ready. Their purpose is to help you, not to overwhelm you. My experiences are similar to what you are going through in your life, and I used these strategies while never giving up to help Max.

As I reflect on our journey, if I had given up, I never would have seen Max play on the basketball team during his junior and senior year. I wouldn't have had the opportunity to present him with the most improved player award that he worked so hard for and deserved, nor would I have seen his happiness at succeeding. It's these small accomplishments in life that make me glad I never gave up on him. I have the memories of our struggles and see how far he has come. His spirit amazes me. We can clearly endure more than we think we can. We had our hard times, and so will you, but we can endure hard times if we apply these life strategies.

I can't tell you when enough is enough, because it is never

enough until you get to where you want to go. I can't tell you how much it takes to get over the hump; just get over the immediate hump, and we will get over the other humps when we reach them. I am always learning, so the journey never ends, but it does get better. The funny thing about life for me is that when I learn something new, I realize how much more there is to learn. It is a lifelong quest. One day, you wake up and try to figure out what you can to help others. Life is not all about you, even when it's going badly, because there are still others wishing they had your small problems. Be grateful, and never give up. Life is full of miracles. You will discover whatever you are looking for. Until you do, keep searching.

Looking back, I know I made the best decision for our family. The investment I made in Max's health has been more than worth it. He has his entire life ahead of him and is well suited to take care of himself. As parents, we never gave up on his health and never stopped investing in his future. I will repeat what I said earlier: the process is hard, which is why every person available must be supportive. Daddies can do so much to make a difference, and we're needed more than ever these days. You have to be firm in life, but still you must be flexible, because life will not always go as planned. Your first step is to decide that you will never give up, no matter what. Decide NOW!

DOS & DON'TS

Do be firm but flexible.

Do what only daddies can do.

Do remember there are consequences for giving up.

Don't ever give up.

Don't ever give up.

Don't ever give up!

CONCLUSION

DECIDE!

"Once you make a decision, the universe conspires to make it happen."
—RALPH WALDO EMERSON

I have had to make some tough decisions in my life, and I am sure you have as well.

After I graduated from high school, I wanted to go into the military, but because I was still only seventeen years old, I needed my parents' signature. They wouldn't sign for me, so I had a make a decision: go to college, get a job, start a business, or rob a bank. Sitting around my mom's house was not an option, and robbing a bank wasn't a good idea.

I didn't have any money for college, so my brother loaned me the money and then showed me how to apply for financial grants and student loans. Since I enjoyed playing football in high school, I decided to go to Troy University and try out for the football team. After a lot of hard work, I made the team—but there were still more decisions to make.

That one decision—to go to college—changed the course of my life. You don't have to go to college to succeed, but you do need to make a decision regarding which direction you would like to go.

As far as I'm concerned, there is only one bad decision, which is to make no decision at all. Decide, and put forth the effort to see your decision through. Life is full of decisions to make, so it helps to learn how to make better decisions.

EMOTIONAL DECISIONS

Whenever it looked like my life was standing still, I reevaluated the decisions that I had made.

After Max was diagnosed with autism, I had to make some emotional decisions. The situation was extremely frightening, because at that time I had no understanding about the condition.

First, I had to make the decision to educate myself about autism, to figure out which information was useful and which wasn't. I had to decide on the best options for Max when it came to helping him reach his fulfillment. I had to decide on a plan of action that included his safety, IEP, medical treatment, physical therapy, and occupational therapy as well as identifying school, state, and private resources and determining which were available to my son.

One of the biggest decisions I had to make was how to pay for everything he needed—and find the time to do it all.

At that time in my life, I was financially stable, without a care in the world. However, I decided I would use my savings, my retirement funds, and a second mortgage on my house to pay for whatever Max needed. It was a very stressful time. I had to ask, "Do I store up all my riches for tomorrow, or do I invest in Max's future today?"

This decision would leave me financially burdened for years to come—but I easily made it to invest in Max's future, and I have never looked back.

A JOURNEY BEGINS WITH A SINGLE DECISION

Some of the earlier decisions I made in my life definitely prepared me for this journey.

For me, it was a good decision to go to college and try out for the football team, because I received a scholarship that paid for most of my schooling. A few years later, our team won the National Football Championship, and I went on to earn a master's degree. It felt like the entire universe conspired to make my dreams come true.

My life has been this way for as long I can remember. I'm not saying it comes easy, but success does come if you make the decision and put forth some effort.

As I moved from college and into my law enforcement career, I continued to face decisions. I decided to become a federal agent because I wanted to help others have a safer life. During my career, I took an oath to uphold the Constitution and to defend it against all sworn enemies. And at twenty-four years old, I had my dream job as a federal agent.

I feel that the entire universe is continuing to conspire to help me help others. I know it will do the same for you.

I now have the opportunity to consult and train others on keeping their children safe because of my twenty-eight years in federal law enforcement. I have been trained by the best and had the opportunity to work with law enforcement all around the world. I have worked internationally in the Middle East, Africa, and South America. I have worked in Chicago, Arizona, St. Louis, and Miami. All of my experience has helped me teach my son how to be safe, and I have trained other parents and law enforcement officers about how to keep their families safe as well.

MY MOST IMPORTANT DECISION

The most important decision that our family ever made was to allow our greatest crisis to become our greatest miracle.

We made a decision and commitment to Max's health and future, as well as to the other people we share our knowledge with.

God's plan for us wasn't to give up on our child. When we made that decision, we also made a commitment to do whatever it took to allow him to reach his fulfillment. There was no way I was going to allow one doctor or 10,000 doctors tell me to give up on my son. When I committed to helping him reach his fulfillment, there was no turning back and no giving up. I would follow through on getting him the best care that we as parents could provide. Our journey wasn't about my ego and trying to make our son into what I wanted him to be, but to give him an opportunity to be what he decided he wanted to become.

I very much wanted him to achieve his dreams.

A few months before his high school graduation, Max and I

were having a conversation. He nonchalantly mentioned that he received a special honors award for three semesters in a row. I told him, "Son, I am so proud of you, and I love you."

I am truly amazed by what an awesome job he has done at adjusting to life in Ecuador, loving school, presenting lectures in front of his classmates, and taking such a heavy course load his senior year while still playing high school basketball and volleyball.

Autism 2 Awesome is a mindset, and every day I wake up thinking about how I can help with Max's safety, education, future, and contribution to humanity. I fall asleep thinking about how I can share with others what I have learned along the way.

My journey started with the commitment to be better than my best, and it continues to this very day through deciding never to give up.

YOU CAN MAKE THE BIGGEST DIFFERENCE

You, too, can decide to put forth your best effort.

I have volunteered and coached the varsity basketball team in Ecuador since 2017. I always emphasize to the players that they need to give their best effort. The best-laid plan in the world is no good if you don't put forth your best effort.

When Max was first diagnosed with autism, it was difficult to grasp the severity of his condition and what it would take to help him reach his fulfillment. But we made the decision that, whatever the outcome, we would put forth the effort.

I really didn't have time to complain, because I was busy working hard, and I believed this hard work would one day pay off. There were plenty of days when I came home and just wanted to rest or veg out in front of the TV—but that wasn't going to help Max reach his best potential. So, even if I was dog-tired when I got home, I had to find a way to refuel, because he and his future were depending on the decisions I made.

I tell everyone I can that the most important step is to start, because it will be you who makes the biggest difference in your child's life.

BE FIRST 2 CELEBRATE, TOO!

In the beginning, I made the decision to "Be First 2 Respond" by setting small, achievable goals for Max for me.

To tell you the truth, I didn't know if I believed I was capable enough to help him. But I did know that I was damn determined to do my very best. So I used my journal and wrote down small, specific, accomplishable goals for the week.

For example, I am a big proponent of sports and physical fitness as beneficial for all children. I would take him outside to the park to dribble the basketball twenty times with his right hand and then twenty times with his left hand. Then, we would attempt to dribble without making a mistake, then without looking at the basketball, then while he was walking, and finally while counting, walking, *and* not looking at the ball.

Then I would help him do pull-ups on the bars in the park. After we reached a certain number of pull-ups, I would encourage him to do at least one more, then another one, and another one. Afterward, I would tell him how proud I was and that I loved him. In these moments, I would tell him that life would get hard sometimes, which is when we have to put forth more effort.

Not only did I make the decision to write these goals down in my journal; I also visualized them in my mind. I actually saw myself playing basketball with Max and sharing story time and "tickle time" together.

Whatever you make a decision about, be sure to write it down. Picture doing it in your mind—and then put a whole lot of effort into getting it done. See your child making strides day after day and week after week. You will be amazed by the results at the end of the week, month, and year.

Take the progress one step at a time. Learn to let go and not be so serious. Build loving memories with your child. Celebrate life, because someone out there has it much harder than we do.

I made the decision to "Be First 2 Respond" and celebrated the tiniest goals that Max and I accomplished. I never wanted to be that parent who berated my child for not being an overachiever. We would talk about what he did right and what we could improve on.

As he got older, I asked him, "How can I be a better dad?" because this position didn't come with a daddy's manual! He talked to me about what I could do better, and I explained to him that I would do my best. Sometimes, I did better; other times, he just figured I was how I was. Children can adapt better than we think they can.

I did my best not to hinder my son's growth because of my imperfections and insecurities. This balance is difficult to achieve with any child, let alone one with special needs. During his early years, we experienced a lot of stress. Looking back, I see why it's so important to celebrate the small victories—because if you don't, you may never see the larger ones. If you can't celebrate, breathe, and enjoy the small things in life, how will you recognize your miracles?

I do my best to find something to be thankful for every day. It has made a huge difference in my life and my attitude.

Take time today to celebrate your first week on the job, your first date, your child's first words, or your child's first smile. Celebrate life because it's worth celebrating.

TAKE ACTION NOW!

I challenge you to choose any one of the strategies from my book and use it for just one day. Why one day? Because that's all it takes for you to start changing your life. You just have to decide and then start. Then on the next day, I want you to use the same strategy to continue changing your life, and when you are ready, choose another one and keep the change going.

I invite you to join our Autism 2 Awesome community by following us on Facebook, Twitter, LinkedIn, Instagram, and YouTube, all under the name autism2awesome.

You can send an email to support@autism2awesome.com to receive a free consultation and learn more about our digital courses. Please contact us if you would like to receive training for your company or organization. I am also available as a guest speaker.

Remember to visit our website at Autism2Awesome.com, and you can purchase my book on Amazon.

Thank you for sharing this information with others who need it.

EVERY ENDING HAS A NEW BEGINNING

We have reached the end of story, which is the beginning of a new story for you and me. Every day can begin a new start. I hope you've gained knowledge that you didn't have before reading this book.

I am grateful that you allowed me to share my journey with you. This process has been very therapeutic for me. During my family's most difficult challenges, I didn't have many opportunities to think about my own emotions. While writing this book, I discovered that I still had some feelings bottled up inside, and I was finally able to breathe and relax, because I know Max is going to reach his best potential.

Thank you all for being such a blessing to me. I hope this book has been a blessing to you. I know that I am blessed, and I give the entire honor to God. He has blessed me, and now I see my greatest crisis became my greatest miracle. He will do the same for you.

Miracles happen every day, and your miracle is just waiting to happen.

I showed up every day for Max, and now the hard work and all the prayers have paid off.

On June 1, 2019, he graduated high school with honors. He has worked hard for what he has accomplished, and he has taught me a lot. I am happy for him and know that he has a great future ahead of him. Today, he is preparing for college and beyond.

I am grateful for the journey, memories, and knowledge I have gained. I have so much, and I am prepared to share life strategies with other families who are caring for someone with autism.

Along this journey, the road twists and turns in many different directions. At times, there seems to be no light ahead, but we never lose hope and we never give up.

Thank you for being so kind and traveling with me from Autism 2 Awesome. Remember to allow your greatest crisis to become your greatest miracle.

With love and appreciation for you all,

KERRY L. BROOKS

ACKNOWLEDGMENTS

I give the entire honor to God.

This book is dedicated to my parents, David L. Brooks and Mary M. Brooks. My father taught us strength, and my mother taught us love. My mom is the rock of our family.

I am grateful to have a wonderful and patient wife in Chauna, who has blessed me with four AWESOME boys, Darce, Xavier, Jansen, and Zaire. My wife has always loved me for me, in good times and bad. She is a truly good woman and a dedicated mother, and she has a heart full of love. I am grateful to all my sons, and they mean the world to me. To be honest, I have a wonderful group of people around me. We share love, and I call all of them family.

I am grateful for Milena, Max's mother. She was the catalyst in starting the healing process for our son and is an incredible mother. I am forever grateful to Max for all that he has taught me and for all that he continues to teach me during our journey together.

I am grateful for Dr. Bruce Shelton. He helped to change the course of our lives toward a brighter future.

I am grateful for my siblings: my sister, Trish, and my brothers, Don, Tony, Glenn, and Norris. My family is the absolute best and also includes all the Brookses and Flakes from my hometown in Alabama. Thank you for my childhood memories.

I am grateful to all my sisters-in-law for marrying my brothers, so Mom didn't have to worry about them. Thank you, Nacoal, Diane, Lisa, and Jeanette.

I am grateful for all my nieces and nephews. Continue to strive forward and be your best.

I am grateful for Linda P. and Sharon B. They have been my investor angels and provided me with awesome friendship and financial blessings so that I could continue developing Autism 2 Awesome.

I am grateful for the love that is shared among our family and friends in Chicago.

To all of my friends who I didn't mention by name, I love you all. All of you have blessed me into and helped me become the person I am today. Thank you for your prayers, your friendship, and a lifetime of memories...what an AWESOME gift to have all of you in my life.

Finally, I am grateful to everyone at Scribe who guided me through the process of writing my book.

ABOUT THE AUTHOR

KERRY L. BROOKS has worked in federal law enforcement for nearly thirty years, also serving as a diplomat during this time in various countries. His most important roles, however, are those of father and husband.

Kerry graduated from Troy University in Alabama, where he was part of a national championship football team. As a proud father of five, he and his wife have dedicated themselves to finding the best strategies for raising their family.

Made in the USA
Columbia, SC
08 December 2023

27330421R00133